Understanding Dissociative Disorders

A Guide for Family Physicians and Healthcare Workers

Marlene E. Hunter, MD

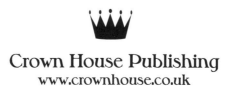

Crown House Publishing
www.crownhouse.co.uk

First published by

Crown House Publishing LtdCrown Buildings, Bancyfelin,
Carmarthen, Wales, SA33 5ND, UK
www.crownhouse.co.uk

and

Crown House Publishing LLC
6 Trowbridge Drive, Suite 5, Bethel, CT 06801-2858, USA
www.crownhousepublishing.com

Originally publishing in hardback (ISBN 978-190442424-6)

Transferred to digital printing

British Library of Cataloguing-in-Publication Data
Acatalogue entry for this book is availablefrom the British Library

13 Digit.ISBN 978-184590050-2

LCCN 2009931261

Printed and bound in Great Britain by
CPI Antony Rowe, Chippenham and Eastbourne

*To Redner, with love and unending gratitude
for your support.*

Contents

Acknowledgments

My deepest appreciation to all my patients, especially in those early years of struggle, who taught me what I had to know about dissociative disorders. You are a wonderfully courageous bunch of people.

Also I want to thank Betty Jo Critchfield for her help with the references; you saved me endless hours of work and did a much better job than I would have.

Introduction

How Did I Get Into This? or, What's a Nice Girl Like You Doing in Such a Psychotherapeutic Minefield?

I saw my first dissociative patient (at least the first one that I recognized) in 1977.

I am a family physician. I had become very interested in the medical and psychological uses of hypnosis in 1972, and within five years it had become a routine part of my everyday practice. When a colleague phoned to say that she was moving out of town and asked if I would accept one of her patients ("I know you're not taking new patients, Marlene, but this woman really needs you"), I agreed.

Thus began a journey that never in my wildest imaginings would I have anticipated—a view into the inner world of the highly dissociative patient. Slowly, I realized that I had another such patient in my very own family practice, and yet another.

She was a pleasant and intelligent patient, and I liked her immediately. In her late twenties, she had a very responsible job in the government offices, which she did well. However, she drove me to distraction, because I never knew where I was at with her. She suffered from terrible headaches; I would prescribe the newest pharmaceutical miracle, she would phone me from work and say, "That medicine is wonderful—why didn't you give it to me earlier?" And then, three hours later, she would be sitting in my office and when she saw me would glare at me and say, "What did you give me that crap for? It isn't worth the paper it's printed on!"

I will call her Jayere, because that is the name I have given her in various papers that I have presented.

Jayere had a documented history of early child abuse. My colleague had done some hypnosis with her and taken her (in hypnosis and at the patient's request) back to a birth experience, in which Jayere reported that she had heard her mother say, "Take the little bitch away."

Now, whether that really happened is not the issue. The issue is that this is what she believed, and if that is how one believes one has been greeted on entering this world, it doesn't bode well for one's future emotional harmony.

In fact, the birth mother deserted the child and the husband when Jayere was three weeks old. The husband, not well educated and in a laboring job, with absolutely no knowledge or experience of children let alone a weeks-old baby, passed her around to various friends so that he could go to work. Ultimately, at the age of thirteen months, she was found on the beach, wrapped in news-paper and left for dead, having been hit in the head with a beer bottle. Bits of beer bottle glass were embedded in her tiny scalp.

She was in several foster homes over the next few years and, at the age of five, was adopted into a family where (as she told me) strict discipline was the order of the day.

As our doctor—patient relationship became established and grew, I became more and more confused. She had had, from previous family doctors, twelve psychiatric referrals. These resulted in twelve diagnoses. I made the thirteenth referral, and thus she received the thirteenth diagnosis—that she had a neurological disorder, not a psychiatric problem. The neurologist, however, said in no uncertain terms that she had a psychiatric problem, not a neurological disorder, although he could not account for the fact that on two separate occasions she had had two distinctly different EEGs.

One day, some months after she had come in to my practice, I was at an American Society of Clinical Hypnosis meeting, where there was an opportunity to discuss problem cases with one of the older physicians or psychologists. Serendipity found me with a psychiatrist from California, Dr. Donald Schafer, who listened very carefully and asked some pertinent questions. Finally he leaned back in his chair and said, "Have you ever thought of multiple personality disorder?"

I'm sure I blanched. "No," I croaked.

"Well, I think you *should* think about it. She has all the criteria."

So I thought about it. And did nothing. And then, several months later, at another hypnosis meeting, I was listening to Dr. Jack Watkins talking about "MPD" (as it was called then) and I said to myself, "Marlene, why are you refusing to believe your own eyes and ears? He is talking about your own patient."

So, with gritted teeth and feeling scared stiff, I gathered all my courage together at one of my next meetings with Jayere and asked, while she was in hypnosis (we were working on relieving the headaches), "Is there any other part of you who would like to come and speak with me?"

And this entirely different voice gruffly said, "Of course! What took you so long?"

What does "dissociative disorder" mean?

In essence, dissociative disorder means an incredible ability to compartmentalize one's mind—but to the point where, in the adult, it often becomes dysfunctional rather than useful.

The term "multiple personality disorder" did a great injustice to the field of dissociative disorders, in my opinion. Although coined with the best of intentions, it was flamboyant and melodramatic and, as we now know, wrong. Dissociative patients do not have multiple personalities: they have a personality structure that is separated into neat little categories and therefore compartmentalized. My metaphor is of a post office, with many post office boxes. Some of the boxes are closed, some locked tight, some with doors ajar—but there is *only one post office*.

The new term, *dissociative identity disorder*, is more accurate—and less pejorative. Many patients have all, or almost all, of the post office boxes open: it is then termed DDNOS—*dissociative disorder not otherwise specified*. The terminology alone is enough to send you screaming in the opposite direction.

The professional jargon for my "post office boxes" is *ego states*. We all have ego states: I explain to my patients that I am a slightly different person sitting here in the office than I am at home, different as a wife than I am as a mother, different in the lecture hall than when I'm enjoying myself with my friends. It's normal. I'm lucky, however—all my ego states know each other so all the post office boxes are wide open; indeed, there are only little screens between them instead of metal walls. It is when there are amnesia barriers between the ego states, so that they do not know each other, that we have a true dissociative disorder.

We used to think that all dissociative disorders were the result of severe emotional, sexual, or physical childhood trauma, especially when the child was very young and the trauma was ongoing, and it is sadly true that that is very often the background. However, there has always been the occasional patient in whom we have not been able to attribute the dissociative symptomatology to such a history. Such anomalies have ultimately led to a whole new understand and basis: the *attachment theory*, first described by Dr. J. Bowlby (1969).

This theory proposes that some children, as very tiny babies, do not have the warm experience of learning a sense of positive attachment—in other words, they have a less than perfect sense of security and trust—to the primary caregiver, who is usually the mother. Instead, they may grow up being somewhat ambivalent about it, or even avoid issues that would demand that the mother show her emotional reliability. This does not necessarily imply abuse, or neglect. It could be that the mother is suffering post partum depression, for example, or her husband is going off to war, or the baby itself is in the hospital, or any one of many other possibilities where there is an interference in the normal

Figure (i): Attachment relationships and the formation of a cohesive identity

- A **cohesive relationship** and the **unity of consciousness** are not automatically achieved. They are **developmental** achievements.

- At 12 months, the child has developed separate emotional states.

- At 18–24 months, one begins to see the blending of emotional states and the development of **megacognitive capacities**.

- These capacities depend on development and maturation of the **orbitofrontal cortex** and other prefrontal areas which concern megacognition.

- Development of the orbitofrontal cortex is **directly related** to the quality of the attachment relationship.

deep connection between the very small child and his or her nearest source of security and—one hopes—love.

With such an unreliable attachment, the emerging child is extremely vulnerable to any subsequent trauma—emotional, physical, or sexual—in his or her environment. When such trauma happens early in life, in the first five to eight years, then dissociative identity disorder may ensue because the child needs to keep things so orderly in his or her young mind that different parts of the personality structure become specifically identified to deal with whatever response is required. On the other hand, such may not be the obvious result but something akin may emerge years later, such as post-traumatic stress disorder (PTSD) among soldiers, or victims of rape or hostage taking or other disasters. In such situations the child escaped the rigid compartmentalization but is still very vulnerable to overwhelming trauma.

What does the personality structure look like?

In the highly dissociative patient, there will always be several typical ego states. There is one that appears to the outside world—some people call this part the "host". There are also, in my experience, at least two others: the Child, and the Angry One. There will also be one or more protectors.

This is not hard to understand, when the history is of abuse and it took place throughout the early childhood years. Child ego states are usually shy, loving, and frightened. They search for what they longed their lives to be—one in which they are unconditionally cared for, nurtured and protected. Because their lives were *not* what they longed for them to be, there may also be the Bully, the Aggressor, the Punisher. Although they may be harder to understand, these latter ego states are often the protectors of the system—because protecting the system, which seems ludicrous to an outsider, gives consistency to their inner world.

On the other hand, the abuse that they endured, be it physical, sexual, or emotional (can you imagine physical or sexual abuse wherein there is *not* also emotional abuse?), was a grave injustice and that is the source of the Angry One. Children are not supposed to be angry, especially at their parents or family, or friends of the family, or other caregivers. If they do exhibit anger, they are often punished. This anger then gets pushed out of sight, but *not* out of the *subconscious* mind, although it may be out of conscience awareness in those patients at the far end of the spectrum. Angry ego states are also among the protectors, because they are exquisitely aware of possible further trauma and may do whatever seems necessary, including expressing rage, to avoid it. The perception of the possible trauma may be off base—far more "possible" than probable—but the protection is there.

As the child grows, other ego states emerge to take care of difficult situations: the one who goes (or went) to school; the one who goes to work; the sexual participant; the one who abhors sex; the one who copes with pain; the wife or husband, the mother, the artist, the whore, the one who deals with going for a job interview, the one who is writing his/her PhD—the list can be very long and of course, includes ego states appropriate for male patients.

You will have recognized, perhaps, that the ego states are connected to emotional states. Often they appear to be simple raw emotion, without connecting that emotion to whatever else is going on, including pain or other physical sensation, intellectual knowledge, or behavior. This is the source of the "BASK" model of therapy proposed by Dr. Bennett Braun in the early 1980s and published in 1986. BASK refers to *behavior, affect* (emotion), *sensation* (physical feeling) and *knowledge*. Reuniting all aspects of the BASK for any given situation, so that the situation itself is complete in its recognition, is an important part of psychotherapy (which may not have much to do with the family doctor but *may* affect the patient's mood, ability to cope, and so on).

Achieving that reunification of remembered experience is a lot harder than it sounds. It almost always requires the involvement and cooperation of several different ego states, each of which holds one aspect of the memory. However, to make you a little more comfortable, remember that it is usually the work of the psychotherapist, not the family doctor.

There are some typical phenomena that will be useful for you to recognize.

Of these, picking up the minimal cues of switching (from one ego state to another) may be among the most useful. Ego states, after you get to know them, will present different manners of speaking (soft, gruff, strident, polite), a different body posture, somewhat different facial expression, which is difficult to describe, different voices (not quite the same as different manners of speaking)—the voice of a child, or a male (in a female patient) or of one who is self-assured or, on the contrary, frightened.

Switching often occurs very quickly, within seconds; on the other hand, sometimes it evolves over several minutes. There is usually a physical clue—a tic of the facial muscles, a hand briefly touching the face, a change in the eyes. After a while, one gets to notice these things automatically. You may or may not have the kind of relationship with your patient that allows you to openly acknowledge the switches. Don't push it, but it's a positive thing if it happens.

Cutting or any other kind of self-harm is not uncommon with dissociative patients. Indeed, such behavior may give you a clue that they are dissociative. For as yet unknown reasons, dissociative patients usually heal very quickly and without infection, even when, for example, the instrument used for self-harm could not have been sterile.

Family members, friends, or workmates may speak of erratic mood changes for no apparent reason.

From the family physician's perspective, there are some clues that may alert you to the possibility that your confusing patient may be dissociative. Some of these are:

- the "thick-chart" patient
- somatization
- frequent surgeries, or requests for same
- confusing lab results
- confusing response to medication
- that the patient "seemed different"
- allergies that seem to spring up from nowhere, then disappear
- self-harm

There may be hospitalization issues:

- surgery
- anesthesia
- pain relief
- childbirth
- trauma/the emergency room
- psychiatric hospitalization
- the importance of communication with consultants

There is symptomatology in virtually all of the physiological systems. Some examples are:

Eye/ear/nose/throat:

- allergies
- visual disturbances
- mouth pain, ulcers
- choking or choking sensation
- erratic deafness

Respiratory/chest wall:

- asthma
- frequent upper respiratory infections
- chest wall pain
- air hunger

Cardiovascular:

- dysrhythmias
- tachycardia
- erratic blood pressure
- severe palpitations
- cardiac anxiety

Gastrointestinal:

- eating disorders: anorexia, bulimia, obesity
- nausea
- unexplained sudden vomiting
- irritable bowel syndrome
- colitis, regional enteritis
- constipation/diarrhea
- abdominal pain not yet diagnosed (NYD)

Genitourinary:

- sexual dysfunction: decreased libido, severe sexual aversion, dyspareunia, vaginismus, erectile dysfunction
- pelvic pain NYD
- irritable bladder
- amenorrhoea
- other menstrual disturbances

Musculoskeletal:

- pain
- unexplained soft tissue swelling
- spasm
- altered gait
- dysmorphia/disturbed body image

Central nervous system:

- seizures (temporal lobe)
- pseudoseizures
- tics and twitches
- tremors (non-Parkinson)
- "coma"—unresponsive collapse "for no reason"

Endocrine:

- thyroid
- sexual hormones, male and female

In other words, practically everything!

I will address many of these issues in the following chapters. We will also look at problems such as boundaries and limits, trust and rapport, how to deal with special favors and gifts, keeping appointments (or not), and walking the tightrope between giving good care and getting overinvolved.

Although it seems incomprehensible to those of us who work in the field, there are many detractors who assert that there is no such thing as a dissociative disorder, that they are a figment of the therapists' imaginations. This is asserted in spite of the fact that the diagnosis has been part of the official psychological/psychiatric diagnostic manuals for more than twenty years, both in North America and other countries through out the world.

In the past decade, a vigorous determination to uncover the true factors in dissociation has led to an elegant and highly sophisticated body of research, and a robust literature. Some of this research will be discussed briefly at the end of this book. It leaves no doubt as to the legitimacy of the diagnosis.

Dissociative disorders are not new. They were described in the literature two hundred years ago. We are simply able now to put them into a more understandable perspective.

Our role

How does this impact on family physicians and other healthcare workers?

We are—or should be—the sentinels. Into our offices come hundreds of patients, and we get to know them, and get to know the families. We see the discrepancies, the unexplained and unexplainable symptoms, the distress and, often, the agony. Most of us would not choose to be the primary therapist, and rightly so; but, with good therapy, most dissociative patients improve, some completely, some at least to a much higher level of function.

When we take our role as sentinels seriously, then our patients can reap the benefits with early diagnosis, appropriate referral and good, knowledgeable therapy, and thus the opportunity to have full and rewarding lives.

Chapter One
The "Thick-Chart" Patient

I was late getting to the office because of an emergency at the hospital, and the waiting room was full when I arrived. Generally my patients were pretty sanguine about waiting, because my receptionist would always explain the reason, but this day there was one glowering at me. Oh, no! I thought. Not *her* today! Mrs. J. was a frequent occupant of one of my waiting room chairs. She seemed to have an endless backlog of complaints, which usually started, "Oh, Doctor, last time I was here I forgot to mention …" and went on from there.

To be fair, she had legitimate complaints (as I described them to myself) because she had been in a nasty motor-vehicle accident two years before, suffering a miserable whiplash, and her husband had advanced emphysema and required a lot of her time and attention. Nevertheless, there were days when I felt my patience slipping as I listened to yet another list of complaints, most of which I could do nothing about—the pollution in the air, the full story of the accident, the fact that her children never lifted a hand to help her. All of these contributed to whatever the symptom of the day might be. Often the problem was poor sleep, or the latest medicine for pain didn't help, or she thought she was getting another cold, which might perhaps turn into the flu. And she always took it as a personal insult if I was late.

What does "psychosomatic" really mean?

How often have *you* looked at your day sheet, on entering your office, and had a pang of tension or a groan of "Oh, no! Not *her* today!"

One of the many burdens that dissociative patients have to bear, is being labeled "psychosomatic". Too often this results in

1

acrimonious relations with their medical caregivers, a sense of great injustice and much anger in the patient, inappropriate referrals, polysurgery, too much and too many prescriptions (often useless or worse than useless), multiple and overlapping lab tests, and numerous other errors of commission or omission as we do our best to navigate the stormy waters.

But remember: "psychosomatic" just means mind-and-body, and everything is psychosomatic because we are not disconnected at the neck: anxiety is reflected in muscle tension; pain is reflected in emotional distress.

Our groans come from frustration—at not being able to decipher the root of the patient's problems or his or her apparently disproportionate reaction to them.

The patient's groans come from the other side of the same coin— "This person's supposed to know what's the matter with me! That's her *job*! Why can't she just get on with it and get me *better*? Instead of that, she sends me for all these tests and makes me spend all that money on useless medicine and then tells me that it's *all in my head*!"

Teeth-clenching abounds.

As a matter of fact, the recognition of a thick chart, and one that seems to be getting thicker with every passing month, ought to alert us that something is obviously amiss here. Allow that little voice (groan) to whisper to you that here there might be an opportunity to do some serious delving and re-evaluating. Then sit down with the chart, pretend the patient belongs to someone else ("I wish!" you might hiss in response), take two and a half minutes to do some self-calming, and start going through it from the beginning.

Look for inconsistencies—in descriptions of the problem, in the consultation reports from your favorite witch doctor(s), in lab results, in other investigative procedures, in response to medication, in what seemed so terribly important (from the patient's perspective) yesterday but seems to be forgotten or dismissed today.

Take particular note of any little messages you may have put on the chart. When I realized that I had another dissociative patient in my practice, I reread her whole chart and sat there, stunned, as I found (in my own inimitable handwriting) a note in the margin saying that "she seems like an entirely different person today". Indeed, she did. She had done a home pregnancy test, which was positive, and a brand-new post-office box was opened—a new ego-state formed, one whose job it was to take care of that pregnancy.

There may be occasions when the patient forgets to come for the appointment, or turns up when no appointment has been made but she insists that it was. This is a classic behavior in highly dissociative patients and one that is particularly confusing to the uninitiated physician, especially when the patient is so demanding. How could she have forgotten an appointment? The answer, of course, is that some other ego-state made it. This may have been one of the protectors in the system who felt that something was amiss.

What to do?

If it is a case of a missed appointment, ask if it is still necessary. Remake it, if so; if the patient says "no", make a careful note in the chart to record the event. If she still wants to come, rebook, but with the same notations in the chart. It is all right to comment that there must have been some miscommunication, when the patient is then sitting in your office. Watch for the reaction, using your best noncommittal physician's facial expression and body language.

If it is a case of the patient's turning up and insisting that an appointment was made, see if you can gently get the details of when that was supposed to have happened. Did the patient phone? What time of day? to whom did she speak? Explain that you are just trying to pin down how and where the miscommunication occurred. Again, make careful notes in the chart. Such notes might, in time, form a pattern.

Be aware of the reactions that are triggered in you by your patient's behavior, demands, or unrealistic responses. Countertransference can be an invaluable guide to the root of any problem, and this is certainly true when we are working with dissociative patients. One of the clues that alerted me to the possibility of another dissociative patient in my own practice was the realization of my irritation at some of her behavior patterns: then the light went on, alerting me that perhaps she was like Jayere.

When you put these tidbits of information together, you may have a legitimate reason to consider that maybe, perhaps, possibly, that patient just *might* have a different diagnosis—one that answers a whole lot of confusing questions.

Do dissociative patients abuse the medical system?

Several years ago I was given an excellent paper to review on the apparent misuse of outpatient medical clinics by some families. The author hypothesized that these were dysfunctional families, with poor personal and social resources, whose various medical problems were more an expression of the psyche than the soma. In looking for connecting links, he found family disruption and often family violence, unsuccessful employment capabilities, little extended family support (although there might be a fairly large group of relatives), past and present problems with the law, and general lack of appreciation of these factors—on the parts of both the patients and the health care workers. Other similar research projects have been published with similar results. They will be discussed in Chapter Seventeen.

He decided to investigate the families for dissociative tendencies and found a remarkable correlation between the degree of unrecognized dissociative phenomena and the frequency with which such patients presented at the outpatient clinic. Indeed, it was a very predictable and reliable correlation—the more frequently the patient attended the clinic, the greater degree of family dysfunction and the greater the incidence of dissociative tendencies and behaviors in the patient. Unfortunately, to my knowledge this paper was never published, but I felt it worthy of comment.

If we extrapolate from this very nice piece of epidemiological research, we can begin to garner a little more understanding of mind–body communication: when the psyche is in a dysfunctional dissociative state, the body responds with its own separation from a sense of wellbeing and—both parts looking for answers when neither even knows the questions—the plethora of psychosomatic problems bubble up to the surface.

Presto! Our thick-chart patient.

Further research into the somatic aspect of dissociative disorders is being done in various parts of the world. Of particular note is the elegant work being done in The Netherlands by Ellert Nijenhuis and his colleagues. Two questionnaires have evolved from this research, which enjoy an exceptional correlation to a diagnosis of dissociative disorders—the Somatoform Dissociation Questionnaire-20 (SDQ-20) and the SDQ-5. They can be found at the back of his book, *Somatoform Dissociation* (1999).

As physicians, we look for answers to these somatic complaints because we want our patients to be, and feel, well. It is all too easy to make yet another referral, ask for one more set of lab tests, prescribe yet another miracle from the pharmaceutical corporations.

Thus we engage in a balancing act. Of course we want to make sure that we have not forgotten anything, omitted exploring some reasonable possibility, or dismissed a potentially dangerous (or even simply annoying) medical condition. So, all too often, we err on the side of overinvestigating. Beware. Too much is not necessarily better than too little.

I fell into this trap often, in the early years, when I was still such a novice in the dissociation field. I prescribed and prescribed, referred and referred. I am trusting my readers to know that I am not advocating any kind of neglect, but rather a healthy skepticism when the usual routes have all proven to reach such disappointing nonanswers.

Worse than that, we may actually do harm to our patients, especially with the polypharmacy. Many dissociative patients have extremely idiosyncratic responses to medication: some are able to tolerate huge doses with no effect whatsoever (or so it seems); others do well with tiny doses—sometimes only a quarter or even a tenth of the "normal" dose. I am thinking, for instance, of antidepressants. These may be used for depression and/or to relieve chronic pain such as fibromyalgia. Those of us who work with chronic-pain patients know that the usual dose of analgesics is often totally useless, yet, strangely, some conditions, such as fibromyalgia, may respond well to these tiny doses of tricyclics. Based on this, I began to offer some of my dissociative patients these very small doses of antidepressants, or of anxiolytics, with occasional rewarding results.

Furthermore, many of us feel that some medications are often contraindicated in dissociative patients. Hypnotics have no place in the therapeutic protocol, nor tranquilizers. Nor, I often used to think, antipsychotics. I have changed my mind somewhat about the antipsychotics used in very small doses. I will speak more about medication issues in Chapter Four. Of course, various medications may be used quite safely by physician therapists who are knowledgeable about dissociation, but it can be a quagmire for the unaware.

As a general rule of thumb, I think of these problems as "psycho-somatic and somatopsychic issues in trauma and dissociation". For example, I would list the following under the heading "Psychogenesis":

● panic attacks
● flashbacks
● sleep disturbances
● derealization
● depersonalization
● vertigo

In the same way, I would list the following under "Somatogenesis":

● body memories
● chronic pain syndromes
● headache
● gastrointestinal disorders

- genitourinary disorders
- air hunger
- eating disorders
- pseudoseizures

These are merely partial lists, of course, but they give an impression that can be useful to put things into a slightly different perspective. Many of these, and more, will be discussed throughout this book in the context of alerting the physician to dissociative expression.

"High-risk" populations

For those healthcare workers who work in underprivileged areas or with high-risk—in the economic and/or social sense—populations, it again behooves us to keep the possibility of a degree of dissociative disorder in the differential diagnosis. At present we have spearheaded a pilot project in the city where I live (Victoria, British Columbia) to evaluate the extent of dissociativity in the "street" population. This project has interested several levels: the tourism groups, both governmental and private; the business community; the public-health offices; the "keep our city clean and safe" groups.

If, as I strongly suspected, the degree of dissociativity is high, then we will have a better grasp of what the problem really is and can get to work putting in place some simple programs, such as opportunities to learn coping skills, problem-solving and life-management strategies, and how to look for and apply for a job. There is already an excellent project for the young street people to take basic job training in janitorial work and in the fast-food industry. It enjoys a spectacular success rate with those who enter the project—about 80 percent. Because there was already a level of trust established, we linked our project with the work-skills project. These projects are funded through several levels of government—local (municipal), regional, and provincial, as well as some community business groups and volunteer agencies that work with those whose homes are on the street. This mini-study was presented at a conference at the University of Victoria (British Columbia) in May 2003. The results were precisely as we had predicted—a level of dissociativity that indicated considerable intrusion into the person's ability to do good problem solving, coping, and decision making. And these were the young people who had enough determination to get themselves into the project.

Local health clinics are also ideal places to begin recognizing dissociative tendencies, which impact on the wellbeing of those patient populations.

I have strayed a bit from the thick-chart patient, but the past few paragraphs seem to fit well in this part of our considerations.

Dealing with crises

From time to time, patients will call or come to the office in a state of crisis. Frequently it does not seem such a crisis to us as physicians or health care professionals. We have to realize that it *is* an emergency to them, and respond with true attentiveness. Use the same skills with which you would respond to any panic attack: speak clearly, in simple sentences. Reassure the patient that you are indeed hearing her. Get her to sit, if possible, and *breathe*. Use some basic relaxation techniques if you can, although she may resist that.

Then, when some degree of settling down has been achieved, you can start to explore, with the patient, what brought on this particular crisis. Eye contact is essential but, paradoxically, be prepared for a shift in ego states, the eyes to drop, the voice or posture to change. These shifts may be minimal but are very important to recognize. Something will have triggered off the response; it is our job to help the patient to find it, and then to discuss, quietly, what could be done about it. The answer may be that nothing can be done about it, so how is the patient going to find the resources to deal with that? I usually point out that patients have been in similar situations many times before in their lives, and somehow they have always found a way to cope. So let us look for the best and most *useful* way to cope.

Remember that patients' coping skills may lie in retreating, injuring themselves, substance abuse, and/or shifting to other ego states. I think it is appropriate to talk about the fact that we all have parts of ourselves that seem better able to cope in a positive way than other parts—for example, there is often a part of us that feels like screaming or running, but that doesn't solve anything; on the other hand, there are also parts of us that can take a deep breath, count to ten, and remember some previous experience that could be an example of a better way to handle the situation.

Dissociative patients are prone to catastrophizing. Nothing seems to be simple, every event is a potential disaster. (Small wonder, given some of their histories.)

Let's take a hypothetical case: Ms. R. She has a long history of a very dysfunctional family and her choice of personal partners leaves a lot to be desired. Nevertheless, she does her best to handle life's exigencies and, for the most part, she manages quite well. Perhaps it might be a situation where you could say, "Do you remember, back a few months ago, when such-and-such happened? If I recall rightly, that was very distressing for you, wasn't it?"

"Yes, I remember. It was awful—I couldn't see any way out of it."

"Yet you *did* find a way through that problem, didn't you?"

"But I didn't do it very well, and I couldn't have managed without—"

Be firm: "*You* were the one who realized that you could do this-and-that, and it worked, didn't it?"

"Well, sort of."

"Yes, indeed. Now, how can you adapt *that* way of looking at the situation to *this* situation?"

"I can't!" (Careful, a wail is developing here.) "They're different."

"Yes, they *are* different, so let's find the areas that have at least some similarities."

You go on from there, being firm, cajoling, reinforcing, giving positive feedback.

"But," you may be expostulating, "I don't have time for all of that. I've got a waiting room full of other patients who deserve my time, too." ("And more appropriately," you may be thinking.)

Well, look at the alternatives. These are situations where twenty minutes spent now may save many hours, house calls, emergency room visits, or office outbursts later. They also offer those little opportunities to wonder about this patient's ego states, if you haven't done so before.

Such scenarios crop up frequently, even when the patient is in a good relationship with a knowledgeable and professionally qualified therapist who truly understands these problems. The family physician is often the link who can hold things together, recognizing when things are going awry, realizing that these symptoms are different—or the same!—and can make appropriate recommendations or observations. These are health issues, and health is our job.

The demanding patient

What about the patient who insists on those further lab tests, another referral, a second opinion?

It is up to us to separate the wheat from the chaff here, and do the professional, responsible thing. At all costs, resist simply dismissing the patient's symptoms; at the same time, ask yourself what might be different from previous similar complaints that might warrant further action. To mix metaphors, it is easy not to see the woods for the trees. Perhaps a second opinion is appropriate.

Most patients will respond favorably to an open discussion of the pros and cons of various options, *as long as they feel that they are being taken seriously.*

We may end up with an angry patient, or an ex-patient. Be sure your clinical records are very clear, with the whole problem well described, what you did and said, your advice, and the patient's response.

Family doctors have the unique privilege of knowing more about the family than any specialist can. We do know what the tenor of the family relationships at least appears to be, always remembering that appearances can be very deceiving, especially in abusive families; we know more about the patient's background, childhood, work record, illness history, susceptibilities, vulnerabilities, and strengths than almost any other professional group.

If you have a thick-chart patient, what are the other charts in the family like? Are they thick, too? Or are they unusually thin? How might you account for those discrepancies, if there are any? By keeping aware that problems in families are seldom isolated to one person, we may be able to head off another problem for a family member, before it assumes major proportions.

To reiterate, when you have a thick-chart patient, look for:

- inconsistencies in lab and/or investigative reports
- a paucity of social/economic resources
- your own countertransference
- multiple referrals and investigations
- polypharmacy
- an apparent crisis one minute, the problem apparently dismissed the next
- forgetting office appointments or turning up when there was no appointment
- questionable family dynamics that you might have picked up
- notes in the chart you may have made (and forgotten) in the past
- the tendency to catastrophize.

Chapter Two
The Emergency Room and Other Critical Situations

She was about sixteen. I was the emergency room doctor the evening she was brought in, with several nasty slashes on her left wrist. There were a few scratches on the right wrist, too, but nothing major.

Her parents were distraught, and said that she had been taking a shower, and then just appeared in the kitchen in her robe, with blood dripping down from her arm. Alarmed, they brought her to the hospital.

She seemed quite indifferent to the whole affair, and looked at her arm, as I was stitching it up, as if it belonged to somebody else.

"What happened?" I asked, as I was putting the bandage on.

"I don't know. I think there must have been a razor blade on the side of the tub and somehow I must have leaned on it." She smiled at me. "Can I go home now?"

"Soon," I said. "I just have to talk to your folks for a few minutes. You can wait by your bed, if you want."

She nodded politely, and went back to the cubbyhole where she had been sitting when I had gone to see her.

I was straightforward with the parents. "It doesn't make sense that she accidentally 'somehow leaned' on the razor blade, which was 'on the side of the tub'," I said. "Those are deep cuts; the blade was held at a sharp angle to her skin and deliberately sliced through the superficial veins in the wrist."

"Are you trying to tell us that she did it deliberately?" the father demanded.

"I'm sorry, but I can't think of any other explanation," I replied.

And that was true at that time. I thought about it often, though, and asked my colleagues if they had ever come across similar injuries with equally impossible explanations. A few had, and we talked about them without coming up with any answers other than the deliberate self-harm.

In those days, I didn't know about dissociation. When I said earlier that Jayere was the first case I had recognized for being what it was, I was speaking the truth. But I must have come across other similar inexplicable histories in the several years that I had been practicing medicine. I have often wondered how many times I had missed the real explanation.

How does dissociation present in the emergency room?

Such injuries, inconsistent with the history, are quite common in emergency wards and it is helpful if the family physician can recognize them for what they are. Self-harm is inflicted by ego states with some agenda that is, in a strange way, meant to be protective: to stop the person from "telling", for example, because, when she was little and she tried to tell someone, she got into more trouble. It may also be a way to "let the pain out" (see Chapter Eleven on eating disorders).

Another frequent presentation is a suicide attempt by someone not thought to be overtly depressed. A variation of that theme is that several people offer different impressions, with a good friend saying that "something seemed wrong", a neighbor saying that she had seen the patient singing as she (the patient) was hanging out the washing, and parents who are just thoroughly bewildered and wondered why their daughter hadn't told them that she was having problems.

At times, a patient will turn up at the emergency room at odd hours, several times over the course of a week or two, having apparently made unlikely attempts to take his or her own life. I am thinking of the patient of a colleague who was found floating in a neighbor's swimming pool, face down, then, a few days later, again admitted because of an "overdose", which was not really borne out by the blood levels of the drug she had supposedly taken. Then there was yet another admission a few days after that with another bizarre story of her trying to throw herself under an oncoming bus, but not throwing herself far enough. It terrified the bus driver, though.

The problem is, such patients apparently recover very quickly from their attempts and are eligible for discharge within a day or so, arrangements having been made for them to see their psychiatrist or psychologist in a few days' time.

It is not hard to understand that emergency room personnel get rather fed up with such patients. Unfortunately, this simply reinforces the distorted belief system of some patients that they are worthless and nobody cares, so they are better off dead. An hour later, such a patient may be having an anxiety attack because the children have been left alone at home and they *need* her.

These are overt examples of the actions of various ego states in a highly dissociative person. One of them (or more than that) has decided it would be better if Betty were dead and has tried to hasten things along. That same ego state does not believe that, if Betty dies, so does the ego state. Ego states in highly dissociative patients absolutely consider themselves to be different people and you cannot reason them out of that belief. (That is part of what the long-term therapy is all about.)

Almost all highly dissociative people have learned never to talk about their inner voices, especially to their doctors and, *extra* especially, never to emergency room doctors and nurses. If they do, they will most assuredly get a needle, and it will also most assuredly, be an antipsychotic. I have already referred briefly to antipsychotics within the context of dissociatives, and this will be discussed in more detail in Chapter Four.

Drug overdoses, not necessarily with suicidal intent, are all too frequently seen. The drugs can be prescription or street, but either way they are a big problem. As we saw earlier, there is something very unusual about the way highly dissociative people metabolize medication. They tend to self-medicate, saving up prescriptions. (In my experience, prescription drugs were far more commonly used than street drugs, but that probably just reflected the population with which I was working.)

Admissions to the psych ward from Emergency are also fraught with potential problems. Psychiatric wards are organized with daily activities in specified time slots. This program works well, generally—except for dissociative patients, whose days (and nights) are not organized around time at all, but around ego-state activity. Consequently, one ego state will attend the anger group one day, and another on another day. The second ego state may not have much, or any, memory of the previous day's group and thus become a source of great frustration for the group facilitator.

Of course, in some areas there are psychiatric units especially designed for dissociative patients and this is quite a different situation. Such units are excellent resources. Nevertheless, dissociative people do best out of hospital, not in it, barring unusual circumstances.

There are several possible scenarios with regard to emergency rooms and family physicians. For instance:

- The doctor is an emergency room physician, full time.
- We are talking about a family physician in private practice.

In the latter case, the family doctor may attend to the patient in the ER herself, or be on call for another physician, or have another physician on call for her.

If you are a full-time emergency physician, take some continuing medical education in dissociative disorders if you can, to further acquaint yourself with the various phenomena. You may find that it provides some answers to otherwise very puzzling conundrums.

If, however, you are a family doctor, you are likely to have at least one dissociative patient in your practice, and more if it is a large practice. The current opinion is that at least 1 percent of the general population has a dissociative tendency sufficient to cause symptoms. Naturally, this does not always mean a full-fledged dissociative identity disorder: dissociative disorder not otherwise specified (or DDNOS) is more common but can be just as difficult to deal with.

Because the problems are usually associated with various crises, the emergency room of any hospital has more than its share. It is a good place to increase your awareness. It also may offer a unique opportunity to speak about these things with your patient, an otherwise difficult subject to pop into the office conversation.

Yet another ER experience is for a family member to bring in the patient, perhaps by ambulance, telling the admitting staff that the patient has been throwing things around at home or otherwise causing mayhem, until it was unbearable and the ambulance was called. The paramedics support this history. Yet when the ER doctor, or the family physician who has been called, goes in to interview the patient, she is pleasant and tractable and has no idea what all the fuss is about. And, shaking his or her head to clear the confusion, the doctor finds the patient's rendition of the history entirely believable. Asking the ambulance personnel whether any medication has been given, the doctor is told, "No".

On the opposite side of the coin, a tractable patient may suddenly begin to raise the roof for no apparent cause.

In both of these cases, a switch has occurred and a different ego state has taken over. Remember that switches can, and often do, occur within a matter of seconds, and sometimes almost seamlessly unless one knows the signals to watch for.

Critical situations

Surgery

Facing surgery is a terrifying experience for a dissociative patient. The idea of being so helpless, especially under anesthesia, is almost more than they can manage to contain. They have nightmares of being sexually abused—there have been too many reported cases of just that scenario—and the lurking mild paranoid response that one finds in some dissociative patients comes to the fore regarding "What are they going to do to me?"; "How will I know what has really happened?"; "Who will protect me?". I do not consider this to be paranoia per se, but rather an overzealous ego state and/or subconscious that is determined to protect the person from harm—a form of hypervigilance such as we see in PTSD. However, it often does sound paranoid to anybody unaware of dissociation. One occasionally also finds, with patients who perceive themselves as having been abused by cults, that they believe a cult member will "somehow" find his or her way into the operating room and "somehow" do some terrible thing, such as managing to plant subconscious suggestions even more firmly in place because of the anesthesia—or even implant a microchip. People who have been severely abused in ritualistic circumstances very frequently do have a schizoid component in their personality structure.

As you doubtless know, intellectual discussion does not dissipate these fears. It behooves us, as their physicians, to do what we can to minimize the fear.

It often involves finding an ego state who can take on some of the management. If you know your patient well enough, you can just ask, "Now, who is the best person inside [remember, to the dissociative patient, her ego states are separate *people*] who can help us with this?" If you are not able to go that far, suggest that we all have deeply hidden resources that we can call on when the going gets really rough and tough, and state firmly that you *know* that she also has those resources. Watch carefully for slight changes in facial expression or eye movement to confirm that she has heard and understood the message.

18

If you are the sort of physician who assists at your patients' surgery, then your reassurance that you will be there to make sure that nothing untoward happens will go far in easing the anxiety. Firmly deal with "Yes, buts".

Because many people who have been abused find touch from another person to be extremely difficult to accept, and because it is inevitable that they will be touched when they are being prepared for surgery (never mind the surgery itself), I offer a suggestion from a patient of mine who used to be extremely dissociative and has two DID sisters and another who is DDNOS (it was a truly awful family). Have the patient write out a list of dos and don'ts to carry with her and present whenever they have to go for surgery, or the dentist, or the emergency room. Such items as "Please never touch me without warning me"; "Please quietly explain what has to be done"; "Please accept tears and a childlike voice"; "Please gently reinforce that you will respect me and my body"; "Please offer some calming time to *breathe* or do some self-hypnosis—a few seconds will do". You can practice presenting such a list in your office by doing a little bit of role play. Your patients will have a more concise list. It's best that they keep the list short, as it is probably going to be accepted by a busy nurse or receptionist or intern or lab technician.

Having blood tests done is one of the most difficult aspect of hospitalization for many patients and some particular reassurance or discussion of coping techniques around that procedure will pay off handsomely for the time spent. Relaxation, visual imagery, and hypnotic approaches are extremely useful.

Surgeons are definitely not in the psychotherapy camp, so do your best to alert him or her as to the complexity with your patient. You may just have to say, "Trust me—this is what it is." Be prepared for head-shaking and disbelief.

Before surgery, either you or your patient's psychotherapist needs to establish that, "Whoever [i.e. which ego state] goes under the anesthesia, comes out of the anesthesia." Many years later I still have vivid memories of one of my patients in the post-surgery ward, glaring at me and saying, "Who the hell are you?" as she came out of the anesthetic and her eyes gradually fixed on my face. It was a young male ego state whom I had not met before. You can imagine the startled looks on the faces of the PAR (Post Anesthetic Room) nurses! In later years, the patient and I chortled over that memory but at the time I felt distinctly discombobulated.

Because surgery is in itself such an invasion, we need to be particularly mindful of the needs of our patients, those who have had both mind and body so often invaded in earlier years. It takes a little more time, but it's worth it—for them, for us, and for rapport.

Obstetrics

All that I described above regarding surgery, applies to women with a history of abuse, who are pregnant and will be giving birth.

Usually the ego system will take care of the situation. I spoke briefly in Chapter One about my patient who arrived after doing a home pregnancy test, who had created an ego state whose job it was to take care of the pregnancy. She literally looked different, and she was. She was diligent about diet and exercise, going to prenatal classes, and doing all the right things to ensure a healthy pregnancy.

When it came near the time for delivery, however, another situation arose. By this time I had recognized the dissociation and together we had talked about several "parts" (at that time it was still called multiple personality disorder). I was therefore caught off guard, but only for a short time, upon hearing a male voice say, "I'm outta here!" when we were discussing labour and delivery. "Fine," I responded, realizing what was happening. "See you in a few weeks." My patient thought it was hilariously funny. "I was wondering what he would do," she giggled. Male ego states have no place in the delivery room.

Being prepared is the most important thing. "Who" is going to deliver, "who" is going to be there in support, "who" will be the mother—not always the one who delivers, I have subsequently found. Your calm acceptance of all these issues will help enormously to keep things on track. Should surgery be expected, such as a planned caesarean section, do your best to explain to the OB/GYN about the circumstances and do the usual preparation for surgical intervention with your patient.

It is even more impossible to avoid touching a woman giving birth than it is to avoid touching a pre-op patient. All the more reason, therefore, to work together and arrive at some agreed-upon strategies. You may be surprised at how responsive the woman is to these suggestions—it is her baby, after all.

(Just a little side comment here. It is not all that rare for a woman to have a distinctly dissociative experience while giving birth. She may dissociate the whole experience, have a psychogenic amnesia, behave in ways totally unfamiliar with her usual style, speak in ways that may have made her blush had she realized what was happening. This is not necessarily linked to pain—in fact, she may completely ignore the pain and that may be part and parcel of the dissociation. I have had a woman in tears, not believing me when I assured her that she had not been given an anesthetic when she delivered; she just didn't remember any of it, from about 7 cm dilated. This has nothing to do with a dissociative disorder—just a dissociative experience in a highly emotional situation.)

Almost immediately after delivery, the Mother ego state takes over—at times, quite aggressively. Not that she's aggressive with the baby—far from it—but she may be aggressive with you or the nurses. Smile and tell her that you know she will be a wonderful mother.

Dental Appointments

This is yet another of those situations where the little list is very important.

Having dental work done is often emotionally excruciating for dissociatives patients—male or female. Usually it has to do with having had oral sex foisted upon them, both giving and receiving, when they were young. The mouth is a very sensitive area of our bodies, emotionally and physically. It has zillions of nerve endings, the sensory apparatus works overtime with taste, touch, aroma and kinesthetic response—that's what mouths are for. However, that is not what mouths are for in some children—or adults, for that matter who are, were, or know that they soon again will be, orally sexually abused.

You can use your common sense as to whether the patient would benefit from a little anxiolytic medication before going to the dentist, remembering, as always, the peculiarities of response to medication in people who are dissociative. Here might be a use for a soothing herbal remedy.

And gently explore the situation with your patient if you can. So often they are relieved to be able to talk about it, especially when they know that they are not going to be disbelieved or ridiculed. In some ways it may be easier if the patient is frankly dissociative—there may be an ego state or two who can come to the forefront and take over the dental appointment, allowing those parts with the disturbing abuse memories to go into their safe place.

The Emergency Room

A visit to Emergency (or Casualty or A & E, depending on where you live) is one more instance wherein that list may be very important. You can prepare the nurses and other clinical staff ahead of time, whenever possible: just giving a short talk on dissociation during rounds is very useful. Forewarned is forearmed, so to speak, so simply talking about dissociation in general terms sets the scene for later visits. Some patients would literally rather die than go to Emergency, because they have been ridiculed or treated badly in the past; others seem to need to turn up there very second week. It is somehow reassuring for them to know that emergency services are available.

To reiterate: dissociative phenomena often manifest in the ER.

Watch for:

- unexplained injury, incongruent with the history
- equally incongruent patient affect
- suicide attempts that somehow seem puzzling
- multiple suicide attempts within a short period of time
- sudden recovery of self-possession
- switching
- overdoses, again incongruent with the situation or history
- complaints from the family with regard to sudden mood changes
- complaints of severe acting-out behavior, but a pleasant, compliant patient
- advise your patients to make a list of the crucial dos and don'ts.

Chapter Three
Contradictory and Confusing Lab Investigation Results

When Jayere first came into my practice I referred her, as I said in the Introduction, to yet another psychiatrist. He was quite sure, after two visits, that her problem was neurological rather than psychiatric and therefore ordered an EEG. It showed an epileptiform blip in the temporal lobe (a not uncommon anomaly in dissociative patients, as I learned later) and he therefore referred her to a neurologist.

The neurologist repeated the EEG and found no such sign. After two visits, he referred her back to the psychiatrist, saying that, in his opinion, the young woman definitely had a psychiatric problem but was neurologically intact.

If there were to be one aspect of dissociativity that causes the most scratching of heads, the disparity in lab results in the same patient ranks high on the list.

Jayere had different EEGs. In many patients, various ego states have different thyroid levels (blood samples taken ten minutes apart), different hematology profiles, different PET scans. These bizarre findings have been reported by many investigators.

In the thyroid study that I undertook, I was looking for a simple test that might give some clue to a possible diagnosis of a dissociative disorder where it was suspected. As people are often sent for blood tests by their family physicians and really don't think much about it, it seemed as if this might be a useful route. Also, I had noticed how many patients either, on the one hand, had a history of thyroid problems themselves or were or had been on thyroid medication, or, on the other hand, whose mothers had had thyroid problems. I wondered if dissociation had something to do with metabolism, because the apparently different physiology of the various ego states indicated that this might be the case. (This was in my first decade of struggling to understand what was then called multiple personality disorder.)

I asked Jayere, and two other patients, if they would agree to be tested, and each woman decided which three ego states would participate: the "host", one aggressive but co-operative alter, and one other of the patient's choosing. My controls were my nurse, my bookkeeper, and me! All the testing was done between 8 and 8:30 in the morning, when each of the various ego states had been present for at least ten minutes.

We tested for TSH, T3, free and total T4, and cortisol.

With only ten minutes between the tests of the different ego states, the results were statistically significantly different. The controls' tests, however, had no significant differences at all, despite our best efforts to "imagine" being a different ego state. I was surprised that, even in the aggressive alters, the cortisol levels were actually much lower than I had expected—a result that I now understand better after reading the research.

Armed with these results, I enlisted the cooperation of several colleagues across Canada and we ended up with fifty cases; sure enough, in all cases, there were statistically significant differences with the various ego states. This study was presented at the 1986 annual conference of ISSMP&D (International Society for the Study of Multiple Personality and Dissociation), as it was then called (now the International Society for the Study of Dissociation, or ISSD).

It was also cited in an excellent article by Miller and Triggiano (1992). The authors described studies on EEGs, visual evoked potentials, brain electrical mapping, sensory phenomena, voice, hearing, endocrine phenomena, allergic responses, specific but different responses to medication, and apparently different withdrawal symptoms between addicted alters and nonaddicted alters in some MPD patients. Many of these reports have not been replicated and badly need to be (including mine), but others have indeed been replicated and many more investigations in the past decade have produced even more convincing evidence that the metabolic/physiological processes of various ego states in a well-differentiated dissociative disorder patient do indeed vary. As I mention in Chapter Thirteen, another of my patients chastised me when I ordered some medication for her vaginal infection, saying "I don't have it, *she* does"—and vaginal swabs taken twenty minutes apart supported her story.

During one of my visits to Cuba, where I have taught regularly for many years, two psychologists asked for my opinion on a young man with whom they were doing some research into the cardio-vascular response to hypnotic suggestions that had emotional content. They were taking pulse measurements on both of his thumbs to support their hypothesis that the content of the suggestion would affect the response. However, they had to stop the procedure, twice. When asked by the young man why they had stopped, he responded to their explanation that the rate was different from one thumb to another by saying, "But a different person lives in the left side of my body than the one who lives on the right side." The two psychologists had not suspected him of being dissociative. Subsequently, they studied several other cases where they did suspect dissociation, and those graphs were subsequently presented at a meeting of the International Society of Hypnosis in San Diego, California.

As family physicians, we have been trained to rely on lab results to help us in diagnosing the patient's problem. When we see such blatant discrepancies in those lab results, we have nowhere to turn for help. However, if we take a deep breath and remember that various ego states can have extremely contradictory signs and symptoms, e.g. one color blind and another not, one needing glasses another not, one being allergic another not—*in the same patient!*—then the disparities simply become one more part of the staggering phenomenology of the dissociative patient.

It does present certain dilemmas, however. Do you treat the lab result? Or the ego state who doesn't have the problem? Do you believe your own eyes? How do you explain it to patients, or their families?

Answer: in a matter-of-fact way.

I believe that it is acceptable to explain to the patient that we have an interesting disparity in the test results. It is appropriate to repeat them, at least once. If you and the patient have an open agreement about the dissociativity, it is not a problem because you can simply discuss this strange aspect of dissociative states.

And so, in a way my hypothesis bore fruit. When there are contra-dictory lab results in the same patient, and when that patient has other aspects that seem to suggest dissociative disorder, the variations may raise your level of suspicion a little higher. You don't make a diagnosis on the basis of contradictory lab results—but you don't ignore them, either.

Chapter Four
Medication

As we saw earlier, I'm not a great fan of medication. However, there are times when it is appropriate (even necessary) and therefore it is important for the family physician to have some understanding of which medications are which.

What works, what doesn't

Let's start with antipsychotics. In general, dissociative patients are very reluctant to take antipsychotics because many of them have had negative reactions to them. This reluctance is not hard to understand: antipsychotics are for psychoses, i.e. to dampen down incoming stimuli and therefore make life tolerable. They work very well in such situations. However, if one dampens down the incoming stimuli for a dissociative patient, it is extremely disturbing because she is used to being acutely aware of minimal cues so that she can keep herself safe. The older pharmaceuticals—the phenothiazines such as chlorpromazine (commercially sold as Largactil), fluphenazine (Modecate), trifluophenazine (Stelazine) and thioridazine (Mellaril)—fall into these categories. On the other hand, I have had some success with very small doses of the newer products, especially olanzepine (Zyprexa), and similarly with very small doses of rispiridone (Risperdol). Quetiapine (Seroquel) has worked well for some patients with PTSD. I would use these products only when the patient was in an extremely agitated phase and then only in very small doses.

We don't really understand why people who are highly dissociative have such idiosyncratic responses to medication, but many (if not most) therapists have concluded that such is the case. I stay entirely away from the dibenzodiazepine derivatives such as clozapine (Clozaril) and very far away from the butyrophenone derivatives such as haloperidol (Haldol). I have occasionally had a patient referred by another physician who was already on medication—I am thinking of one in particular who took Mellaril and seemed to be doing well with it—and I would not make changes in such a therapeutic regime unless the patient became adversely affected. In time, the need for medication almost always diminishes; it seems foolish, especially before one gets to know the patient better, to rock the boat and risk unwanted side effects where none existed before.

But to simplify the wordy paragraphs above, my personal favorites in the antipsychotic realm are:

- none!
- olanzepine (Zyprexa) in small doses
- respiridone (Respirdol) in very small doses
- quetiapine (Seroquel) for PTSD.

On the other hand, there are times when one of the ego states is so depressed that the black cloud envelopes the whole system and nothing gets done. In such a situation I would certainly advise using an antidepressant before the therapy comes grinding to a major impasse. In such situations I almost always choose one of the SSRIs (selective serotonin-reuptake inhibitors) such as paroxetine (Paxil) or sertraline (Zoloft).

I do not like fluoxetine (Prozac) because several patients who were on that medication when they came to me, or for whom I prescribed it at the beginning of my learning curve, suffered terrible nightmares, which disappeared rapidly when the medication was changed. The tricyclics such as amitriptyline (Elavil) have been used for years but are no longer produced in the same formulae, at least not in North America. If patients are on a medication when I first see them and it is working, I don't change it. I don't use clomipramine (Anafranil), doxepin (Sinequan), imipramine (Tofranil) or nortriptyline (Aventil). There are others (bupropion, trade name Wellbutrin, or trazodone, trade name Desyrel) that some physicians have found to be effective. The important thing is to find one that lifts that black cloud so that therapy can continue without undue side effects.

My personal favorites are paroxetine (Paxil)—definitely the favorite of the favorites—and sertraline (Zoloft), for those for whom paroxetine has not produced the desired effect.

Polypharmacy

It is important that all patients, no matter what their particular problem may be, be aware of the potential dangers of poly-pharmacy—i.e. mixing and matching medications and dosages according to what the perceived problem may be at the moment. The possible complications are multiplied several times over with the dissociative patient, or even a patient who has many dissociative features without fitting into the diagnostic categories of dissociative disorders. Part of the reason for this warning is the peculiar way in which dissociative patients meta-bolize medication, which I shall refer to in greater detail a little later.

Although there is a natural wish on the part of both patient and physician to prescribe an anxiolytic when the patient is beside herself with anxiety, usually the anxiety covers a degree of depression and it is more efficacious to give the antidepressant, thus taking care of two birds with one pill. However, see the note on lorazepam, below.

Occasionally, a patient will have pseudoseizures and the need for anticonvulsants is questioned. Of course, the first thing is to ascertain whether these truly are seizures—which certainly need medication—or not. Of all of the various anticonvulsants, the only one with which I am truly comfortable for a dissociative patient is one of the iminostilbene derivatives, carbamazepine (Tegretol). Naturally, I would bow to the wisdom of a neurologist who might feel otherwise (especially if there is any question whether the seizures are "real", because they certainly are "real" to the patient). One of the benzodiazepines, lorazepam (Ativan), is frequently handed out in emergency rooms for a very anxious patient. It works, but tends to be habituating, which is not what we want and may become a further complication.

For the benefit of those who find the chemical sources of these medications fascinating, I have put a more detailed list at the end of this chapter.

As far as hypnotics are concerned, I stay away from them if possible. It is far more useful to encourage using self-hypnosis, or yoga, or some other form of meditative approach.

Peculiarities of medication metabolism

An entirely different problem may arise if the patient has an infection and requires antibiotics, or a condition such as thyroid dysfunction (hypo- or hyper-) or diabetes. Of course, medication is appropriate in such situations but often the patient does not want to take it—or, at least, some parts of the system don't want to take it! I have found the perfect answer: "Well, that's easy. Just let those who need it take it, and those who don't need it don't take it."

And how could that possibly work, you ask?

I haven't a clue. But I do know that, with a highly compartmentalized personality structure, it is often an acceptable solution to the patient, and also that equally often that person seems to need less medication than one would have thought. There is so much we still have to learn about the metabolism, biochemistry and physiology of dissociative disorders.

The subject of pain is discussed in Chapter Five but deserves to be considered here also.

Analgesics are frequently sought after (not only by dissociative patients!) and this is easy to understand. Frequently, the patient does experience terrible pain and almost always "some reason" can be given for the pain. This discomfort could be similar to a type of polymyalgia, or a fibromyalgia, or menstrual pain, or any of the many types of pain that people experience. One type of pain that almost all dissociative patients have, at least at times, is so-called "switching headaches". These headaches are a real enigma, because the neurological sources have really not yet been identified. Because they are so universal in this patient population, they deserve special mention.

One of the questions asked in the DDIS (dissociative disorder interview schedule) concerns having been diagnosed with migraine headaches. One of the reasons that the question is there is because switching headaches are often confused with migraine headaches. They are severe, there is no doubt about that. But they are not vascular headaches: there is no aura, they do not last very long—often just a matter of minutes—and they are not accompanied by nausea, photophobia or the other physiological side effects that so often accompany the true migraine. They do not require medication. In cases where they last longer than normal, simple measures such as an ice pack on the head will relieve the pain very quickly. I usually teach the patient some hypnotic pain-relief techniques, which are often very effective.

It is prudent to be very wary of prescribing analgesics because many dissociative patients have an incredible capacity for them. They may be unbowed by doses sufficient to subdue someone twice their size and half their age. It is a very slippery slope to get onto, so the best thing is to stay away from using them as much as possible. This applies to postoperative analgesia, too. Of course I am not advocating allowing patients to suffer, but encourage them to use their own abilities to relieve pain.

It is also true that occasionally a dissociative patient does far better on tiny doses of medication—doses that we would usually consider to be useless. It is far easier to start with small doses and increase them if necessary, than to start with doses that are higher (or even "normal") and then wonder why the dose is not effective and get into the problem of how much to increase the dose when the real need is to *decrease* the dose.

The best advice is to use medication only when you believe it to be necessary, use as small a dose as is needed to achieve relief, and wean the patient off the medication as soon as it is prudent to do so. In the case of antidepressants, this may mean months or even more than a year; with hormones such as thyroid, or diabetic medicine, titrate it as carefully as you can and monitor at frequent intervals.

Psychotropic medications

Antipsychotics

benzisoxalone derivatives: rispiridone

butyrophenone derivatives: haloperidol

dibenzodiazepine derivatives: clozapine

dibenzothiazepine derivatives: quetiapine

dibenzoxapine derivatives: loxapine

diphenylbutylpiperidine derivatives: pimozide

phenothiazines (aminopropyl): chlorpromazine, promazine

phenothiazines (piperazine): fluphenazine, trifluoperazine

phenothiazines (piperidine): thioridazine

thienobenzodiazepine derivatives: olanzapine

thiozantine derivatives: zuclopenthixol

Antidepressants

nonselective monamine-reuptake inhibitors: clomipramine, desi-pramine, doxepin, imipramine

phenethylamine bicyclic derivatives: venlafaxine

selective serotonin-reuptake inhibitors (SSRIs): fluoxetine, fluvox-amine, paroxetine, sertraline

various: bupropion, nefazodone, trazodone, L-tryptophan

Anticonvulsants

barbiturates and derivatives: phenobarbital, primidone

benzodiazepines: clonazepam, diazepam, lorazepam

iminostilbene derivatives: carbamazepine

various: paraldehyde

Hypnotics

aldehydes and derivatives: chloral hydrate, paraldehyde

barbiturates: phenobarbital, amybarbital, secobarbital

benzodiazepines: alprazolam, bromazepam, flurazepam

cyclopyrrolones: zopiclone

various: valerian root.

This is by no means an exhaustive list, but it certainly covers most of the medications that are currently in use. My caution remains the same: when it is possible to help the patient without using medications, do so; when medication is needed—such as with severe depression, paralyzing anxiety, a very fragile hold on reality—then by all means use the tools that the pharmaceuticals have provided for us. And choose wisely.

Chapter Five
Pain

The next three chapters are about chronic syndromes. For many years I have thought of, and treated, chronic syndromes as if they were a type of dissociative disorder. As the next three chapters evolve, I am sure that you will understand why I take that approach. There are striking similarities between the chronic syndromes and the various dissociative disorders with respect to signs and symptoms, and to neurological and neurophysiological phenomena. Two charts depicting these visually will probably explain it better than the words which I use to describe it. However, words there shall be.

Having said that, in what follows you will also find far more references to the literature than in other parts if the book. It's important to know where the research is focusing. So many chronic syndromes used to be thought of and dismissed as imaginary, or manipulation, or seeking attention, or secondary gain, or "weak-minded". Consequently, it is heartwarming now to find the plethora of good research finally surfacing. Furthermore, there is an effort to connect psyche and soma: as the old song about love and marriage states, "you can't have one without the other".

This chapter dwells on pain, and its various aspects and presentations.

Headaches

Virtually all dissociative patients suffer from headaches. The important thing to recognize is that not all headaches are the same, and that people who are highly dissociative—those with dissociative identity disorder—have a specific type of headache that has to do with the switching process from one ego state to another. So far, no one has been able to explain the neurophysiology of this to me, but it is very common. Apparently it is excruciating, but usually fairly short-lived. It is often one-sided, and very often is misdiagnosed as migraine. It is not migraine—these are not vascular headaches. The trouble is, we don't really know *what* they are.

They seem to be akin to a headache that many people describe after coming out of hypnosis, especially if they are just learning the techniques. Usually the headache itself disappears after a short time—often by the time they get home, for example—and after a few sessions never seem to bother the person again. I think, therefore, that it has to do with a dissociative process itself (as hypnosis is also a type of dissociative process) and not to be feared. However, it can be disturbing for many reasons, one of which is that we don't like to dismiss an excruciating headache. What if it *is* something that needs immediate attention? Usually, the patient himself recognizes the headache and it may become a case of patient's reassuring the physician.

The misdiagnosis is one of the most troubling aspects, from several perspectives: many patients are sure that migraine is what they are experiencing (having been told that by more than one doctor) and are frequently taking medication designed to control vascular headaches. However, there is no aura, no photophobia, no nausea—none of the well-recognized phenomena that do accompany a true migraine. It also may be difficult, in the first stages of working with dissociation, and before good rapport is established around the diagnosis itself, to explain to the patient that these headaches seem, for a significant percentage of patients, a "normal" part of being dissociative. Who wants to hear that, for heaven's sake?

On the better side, the switching headaches also seem to abate as therapy progresses. Assuming that your patient is now well connected to a competent psychotherapist, it is a good idea to inquire about the headaches from time to time. This serves a dual purpose of monitoring how the therapy is going, and reassuring the patient that you are interested in his wellbeing.

The other type of headache to which they are prone is (you will not be surprised to read) tension headache. All the basic criteria are there—the position across the forehead and temples, the tight muscles in neck and shoulders, the tingling scalp, the anxiety. Deal with those headaches as you always would, being very sure to reassure the patient that it is no wonder he is experiencing some tension, and suggesting cold cloths or ice packs, meditation techniques, and whatever else you have in your armamentarium that works. Stay away from medication as much as you can, remembering that dissociative patients often have a strange response to pharmaceuticals.

Chronic pain syndromes

I have written extensively about this in a previous book (Hunter, 1994). Because one particular patient's chronic pain was an elusive type of headache, diagnosed as migraine but years later rediagnosed as "central cerebral pain syndrome", her story overlaps the previous commentary on headaches and the next section on chronic pain syndromes. I shall quote from the opening paragraphs of that book:

> Samantha is an intelligent and articulate 32-year-old with gorgeous red hair and a bright, ready smile. She is a research chemist, very respected in her field. She was referred by her family physician and I asked how I could be of help to her.
>
> "I have migraine headaches," she said. "I have had them for twelve years."
>
> Although she had had headaches from time to time since her teens, it was in her early twenties that they began to intensify. The pain was now so excruciating that she felt that she had reached the limit of her endurance. And it was seriously interfering with her work—she had had to give up on very important project because, with the amount of medication she needed even to keep the pain tolerable, she couldn't think straight.
>
> Early last year, she was admitted to University Hospital for two or three days, because her neurologist wanted to sort out her medications and get her on a better regime.
>
> She was there for four months.

After several unrewarding attempts to subdue the headaches with hypnotic techniques, I decided to use an approach I had not yet tested in such situations: an ego-state approach. My thoughts were based on the common complaint of "I see him [the pain or fatigue and usually identified as male] coming and he just takes over and *I can't do anything about it!*"

That is an extremely dissociative way of describing experiences, and is one that I have heard time and time again.

Now, ego state therapy is a well-known and respected approach in the psychotherapy of dissociative disorders. Why not, then, utilize a similar approach in these chronic disorders that take such a toll on the person's life? The general concept behind my reasoning is that, in such syndromes, various ego states assume a sort of life of their own. Thus one may be able to discern and describe a depressed ego state, an angry ego state, an ego state that represents activities the sufferer used to be able to do, and so on. Identifying these various parts of the person's emotional land-scape forms the basis for using the approach, perceiving each in a positive rather than negative way as contributing to the whole system. It's not really rocket science, and it is extremely adaptable. Besides, the patients are intrigued.

I explained it to my patient and she was more than willing to explore it. Over time, she began to see subtle changes—the headaches no longer controlled her life in the way they had been doing for so long. It wasn't magic, but it was something.

She certainly agreed that she had these parts of herself—a part that was very angry, a part that got very depressed, a part who used to be the life of the party but now didn't even want to *go* to a party, a part that was the research chemist, and several more. And the part that was the Pain, which would come and just take over, sending her whimpering to her bed.

You see what I mean about its being very dissociative in nature. As I read this last paragraph over, I also realized that in one instance I referred to a part by using the personal relative pronoun "who" instead of the impersonal "that". As I say, these ego states take on a life of their own, for the therapist/physician, too.

However, we must not forget that research is providing new possibilities for understanding chronic pain syndromes all the time. Recently, Lidbeck (2002) published an exciting paper about central hyperexcitability as being a factor in chronic musculoskeletal pain. The author wondered whether certain types of chronic pain may really be explained by abnormalities in central pain modulation (which would apply to Samantha). Several years earlier, Crawford (1995) wrote and spoke extensively about hypersentitization of the pain response in chronic-pain patients. The research is enticing; but we still have to work on the front line, with the patients and their fears, hopes and past experiences. (And ours, too.)

I also want to make a special mention here of chronic pelvic-pain syndrome, especially in men. Many people are inclined to relate this syndrome with early sexual abuse and we can understand how that could be related. It also invokes the theory of dissociativity.

Putting that to one side, however, it is important to bring ourselves up-to-date on this type of chronic pain. There are several interesting articles in the recent literature about male chronic pelvic-pain syndrome—usually linked to prostatitis. However, Bjerklund-Johansen and Weider (2002) succinctly state in their abstract that "Patients with non-inflammatory chronic pelvic-pain syndrome ... are characterized by the absence of objective findings". Because there is really nothing to link the symptoms with the prostate or other male organs, researchers were looking to find similarities with interstitial cystitis in women. They are seeking answers in the realm of molecular biology.

Lee et al. (2001), however, focused on the neurophysiology, and concluded that patients with chronic pelvic-pain syndromes have an altered sensation of perineal pain, which is thought to be elicited by heat.

Zermann et al. (2001) feel that a neurobehavioral perspective should be used as we struggle to understand the neurophysiological pathways. They also feel that both causal and symptomatic treatment approaches should be used in order both to influence basic pain mechanisms and to relieve pain as soon as possible.

Because much of the discussion in this book seems directed toward women, I felt that it was important to include these specific references to a syndrome that is frequently found in men. I do think, of course, that similar therapeutic approaches are equally appropriate for both genders. Men have ego states, too.

Fibromyalgia

Fibromyalgia (known by various synonyms in various parts of the world, such as chronic myalgia encephalopathy, or ME) is, even now, when it has had so much media attention and support groups around the world, debated as to whether it is real or "imaginary". I find it hard to think of its being imaginary, since it has such distinct diagnostic criteria, especially with regard to trigger points. There are also research studies using "pain brain scans" and electromyography, which are offering new insights— I'll speak more about those a little further on. Fibromyalgia is yet another example of a chronic pain syndrome.

It is probably one of those entities that are also considered to be "body memories", i.e. the long-term effect of abuse, especially child abuse. Whatever its origins, it is *not* imaginary. Pain is never imaginary: it is real to the person experiencing it. We may not be able to trace the source, but the pain itself is always real. Fibromyalgia intrudes terribly into people's everyday functioning, often rendering them incapable of working, taking care of children, traveling, or having good sexual relations with their partners. It just plain hurts too much.

Several years ago, at an ASCH annual meeting, Ronald Melzack was discussing the gate theory of pain, and went on to explain his concept of a neurosignature, which is very specific for each person and has to do with past experiences and how they are reflected in present responses. When it came time for questions, I wanted my question to be on the tape recording, so I leaped to my feet. "Is it possible", I asked him, "that this could also be what we call body memories?" "Of course," he answered, and a cheer went up in the room.

Figures 5.1 and 5.2 show my graphic way of linking these chronic syndromes to a dissociative type of process. Across the top, we have chronic fatigue syndrome, fibromyalgia, chronic pain syndrome, somatization disorder some types of depression, PTSD, DDNOS, and DID. You can easily see the similarities.

Figure 5.1: Chronic disorders from a dissociative perspective

Signs and symptoms	CFS	FM	CPS	SOM	DEP	PTSD	DDNOS	DID
% in population	3–5%			4%				1–10%
Unexplained body pain	+	+++	+++	++	+	++	++	++
Headache	++	+++	++	++	++	++	+++	++++
Sleep disturbance Stage IV non-REM	+++	++++	+++	+++	+++	++	+++	++++
Nightmares	++++	+++	+++	+++	+++	++++	+++	++++
Fatigue	++++	+++	++	++	++	+	++	+
Psych. Dx's	+++	+++	+++	++++	+++	++++	+++	++++
Neurophysiol. Dx's	++	++	++	++	++	++	+++	++
Hx dysfunction &/or abuse	+++	+++	+++	++++	++	+++	++++	++++
Family dysfunction	+++	+++	++	+++	++	+++	++++	++++

Look particularly at the similarities under "unexplained body pain", "headache", "history of dysfunction and/or abuse", "family dysfunction" and "fatigue". Also, see the neuropsychological similarities such as the "helpless/hopeless syndrome",

Figure 5.2: Chronic disorders from a dissociative perspective

Neurophysiol/ Neuropsychol	CFS	FM	CPS	SOM	DEP	PTSD	DDNOS	DID
Sleep deprivation	+	++	++	+	+	+++	++	+
Distortions in cognitive THOUGHT (3 months)	+	+	+	+	++++	+	+++	+++
Cerebral lateralization to (R)	?	+	+	+	++	+	+++	+++
Helpless/ hopeless	++	++	+++	+++	+++	+	+++	++
Ratio F:M	?	10:1	?	?	10:1	?	?	10:1
Disturbed body image	+	+	?	+++	+	?	+++	++++
Anxiety/panic	+	+	+	+	+	++	+++	++++
Sexual abuse	+	++	+	+++	?	++	+++	++++

and, as time goes by and their suffering seems not only unimproved but getting worse, a quite profound "negative self-hypnosis". They begin to tell themselves that they will never get well, this pain will be with them forever, they'll never be able to work again or maintain a strong personal relationship. In time, if this negative self-talk is not recognized and stopped in its tracks, they begin to fulfill their own prophecy. You have probably seen and heard it from your own patients.

At times I have used Figures 5.1 and 5.2 to point out to patients my theory about chronic syndromes. Invariably, their eyes light up. "Yes!" they say. "That's exactly how I feel. Some other part of me *takes over*! I don't even feel like 'me' anymore. In a way, I've lost myself."

I am not alone in linking fibromyalgia with trauma-spectrum disorders. In a very interesting study (Cohen et al., 2002), the authors found a definite relationship between fibromyalgia and PTSD symptoms (remember "body memories"). In this comprehensive study, the results showed clearly that 57 percent of patients who met the diagnostic criteria for fibromyalgia had clinically significant levels of PTSD symptoms. These symptoms included the well-known responses of hyperarousal, anxiety, flashback-type experiences, and depression. Furthermore, the prevalence of such symptoms in this group of patients was also significantly higher than PTSD symptoms in the general population. Also, women seemed to be more affected than men. The authors concluded that there is a significant overlap between PTSD and fibromyalgia. Another study (Wikner et al., 1998) suggests that the sleep disturbances in FM may be due to decreased nocturnal melatonin secretion. I wonder whether the same might occur with other chronic disorders, and whether that is what also happens with PTSD or dissociative disorders.

Nor are fibromyalgia symptoms solely self-defined. There are now several studies in the literature describing measurable pain signals in the brains of FM patients.

Gerdle (2002), in reporting electromyography studies in fibromyalgia patients, suggests that the reports of "muscle tension" by patients, in describing their pain, does not correlate well with EMG hyperactivity, but more with personality traits such as anxiety. However, the meaning of fatigue and tiredness to patients with fibromyalgia does not seem to be the same as to patients who do not have these syndromes. Women without FM use fatigue to indicate that they need the rest, in order to recover from whatever ails them, whereas women with FM seem to regard their bodies as burdens that they must carry, an intrusion, something getting in the way of recovery. These are very different scenarios. The FM descriptions also seem to me to be a dissociative interpretation— the body being distinctly separate from the psyche.

As physicians, we also must recognize our own role. With fibromyalgia, as well as with other disorders such as irritable bowel syndrome, studies report a distinct difference in the way physicians categorize the patients' reports, from the meaning that the patients themselves intend. We are too quick to dismiss, be skeptical, or moralize. None of those attitudes helps our patients. Perhaps it reflects our sense of helplessness rather than our lack of caring, but you can easily imagine how it could be interpreted by patients in pain.

Suggestions abound as to what can be helpful for these often desperate folk. Certainly, *small* doses of the tricyclics, e.g. amitriptyline, have proven useful. (It was recognizing the similarities between the chronic disorders and dissociative disorders that gave me the idea of using small doses of medication with my dissociative patients, rather than starting with the "normal" dose, and—surprise, surprise!—some of them did quite well.)

Exercise is also important for FM patients, but it is difficult to get that message across to someone who experiences severe pain whenever he moves. One type of exercise, known as Pilates, seems to be particularly useful and is gentle. Many physiotherapists are trained in this technique.

It also seems to be true that the symptoms of fibromyalgia do abate as the person gets older. That suggestion may not be embraced too avidly by the thirtysomething patient, however.

We may also wonder, especially since Ellert Nijenhuis's work, whether all these chronic syndromes are simply variations of somatoform dissociation. I don't know the answer to that. I do know that it is grossly unfair, and just plain bad medicine, to discount them as being "all in your mind"—which equates to "imaginary" for most people.

What can you do?

I would suggest you think about using your own personalized form of ego state talk. Ask your patients whether it ever seems as if part of their pain is almost like a separate entity that comes and "takes over". My bet is that a significant number of them will connect immediately with that suggestion. Then you can use it in a positive way, such as by saying, "So, we're not going to let that part become your whole life, are we?" That way, you are a partner in keeping them strong but it is also up to them to recognize what's happening. And it doesn't in any way imply that you are disregarding their suffering.

It may be that, as time goes by, you and your patient develop sufficient rapport to allow the exploration of several more ego states, having to do with directly describing what it is like for the patient. I am almost sure that there will be an angry part, a depressed part, and a part reflecting interpersonal relationships—son or daughter, parent, spouse. It often helps to invite the various ego states to vent their emotions.

There will also, almost always, be secondary gain. With chronic syndromes, this is so common that it can be considered normal. Therefore, another opportunity for you to do something in a situation where there is precious else that you can do is to explain what secondary gain really means: it is *never* the same as malingering, which is the deliberate intent to deceive. It is, instead, a desperate and mostly subconscious attempt to find some sort of comfort in an otherwise bare, comfortless situation. If one can enjoy a little extra sympathy from a spouse or a friend, why not? The trick is to keep it in perspective.

Smith, Lumley, and Longo (2002) published an interesting paper on what they termed *emotional-approach coping* (EAC). They differentiated this from emotion-*focused* coping strategies, which they termed negative and seeming to be related to worsening rather than relieving the pain. Passive coping strategies (emotion-focused) were associated with more pain, impairment, and depression, whereas emotional-approach strategies seemed to be related to less depression and what they termed "affective pain". My interpretation of their results is that, when used positively, recognizing the emotional component and working psychotherapeutically with it in an active process is helpful, whereas focusing on the emotions of depression and anxiety only deepens the pain. One zeros in on the positive and adaptive emotions and utilizes them rather than becoming further enmeshed in negative affect. This is not unlike recognizing the different ego states and utilizing those that offer strength and purpose.

These same authors (Lumley, Smith, and Longo, 2002) have also published a paper on the relationship of alexithymia to pain severity and impairment in chronic pain patients. They found that alexithymia was moderately correlated with less self-efficacy and greater catastrophizing, and substantially correlated with greater depression. That certainly fits with the clinical experience of all of us who work with chronic pain patients.

One wonders if the above responses could be relieved somewhat by medication, as it suggests a neurochemical element with the depression. Explore small doses of tricyclics. You may catch two birds with one stone, by easing the pain response somewhat and alleviating sleep disturbance. Remember also that Substance P is secreted when the person is sleep-deprived: more pain, less sleep, more pain. What a vicious cycle.

To reiterate:

- chronic syndromes have many dissociative aspects
- chronic pain syndromes include some types of headaches and fibromyalgia
- an ego-state approach may be useful
- secondary gain and malingering are entirely different entities
- there is considerable research into the role of neurological/neurochemical imbalance in chronic pain disorders, which in turn affects the psychological responses
- we are not disconnected at the neck!

Chapter Six
Other Chronic Syndromes

Chronic fatigue syndrome

Chronic fatigue syndrome (CFS) is yet another trial in many people's lives, and yet another instance where the patient is so often accused—implicitly if not explicitly—of malingering or otherwise deliberately seeking sympathy. It is also another instance wherein the dynamics of the patient response are in many ways similar to the phenomena expressed in dissociative disorders. (See Figures 5.1 and 5.2 on pages 43 and 44 respectively.)

CFS has had a stormy history—or histories. During the past five decades, it has been attributed to many causes: mononucleosis/Epstein-Barr virus was a popular culprit during the sixties and seventies; then other viral entities were considered to be the culprits when cases were reported wherein no EBV could be identified; "just depression in another guise" was one that I often heard from my colleagues during the seventies and into the eighties; "somatization disorder," growled some disgruntled GPs throughout the several decades when CFS seemed rampant. Environmental sensitivity was bandied about, as were immunological deficiencies. For some reason, it has not been nearly so frequently diagnosed—at least in my part of the woods—during the past few years.

It is true, looking back at medical history, that each generation seems to have devised its own brand of CFS. Unfortunately, this interpretation does not help the patient.

Twenty years ago, I attended an annual meeting of the College of Family Physicians of Canada (of which I was, of course, a member) and one of the leading speakers was a psychiatrist, Dr. Susan Abbey. She was to give a fairly extensive presentation about Chronic Fatigue Syndrome. I went, fully prepared to be angrily confrontational, as I had had the misfortune to come up against psychiatric colleagues during the previous three or four years who seemed determinedly antagonistic to the idea that CFS might be "real".

She was wonderful. She described how, in her view, there were four aspects to be considered, four sets of symptomatology, each of which may present differently and have different outcomes.

The first situation was a well-defined and well-remembered history of a viral illness that seemed to get better, but then stopped doing so. The patient began to feel more and more fatigue; in time, even getting up out of a chair required immense effort. It usually attacked women—although some men were afflicted too—and usually those from late teens to early thirties. For some reason, it seemed as if the more active the patient had been before the illness, the greater the dysfunction that ensued; a bright vigorous young athlete who usually thought nothing of running five miles was unable to summon up the energy to walk slowly to the bottom of her driveway. Her *short* driveway.

The second group also complained of a viral illness, but it was a much sketchier history. "I think it began it February," one woman told me, "or maybe it was March, and then it seemed to keep on getting worse, but I'm not really sure when it started. I sort of remember feeling under the weather through Christmas …"

The third group, in Dr. Abbey's view, consisted of those whose primary diagnosis was depression and the fatigue followed along with that, rather than *causing* the depression.

And in the fourth group, with absolutely no disrespect implied, were what she called the "walking wounded".

Each group carried a different prognosis: Group 1 would spontaneously begin to improve (really improve) after about 18 to 24 months and would go on to full recovery; for Group 2, the prognosis was less favorable and we would see them get stuck in a mode of dysfunction that could go on for many years. Perhaps you may have had such a patient—ten or fifteen years later, the level of function was marginal at best and the poor patient utterly miserable. (And angry! "Why aren't you *doing* something?" is what she is dying to say—but is afraid to, because it is dangerous to upset your doctor. What would happen if that doctor told you to get another physician?)

Naturally, the appropriate diagnosis of depression required the appropriate antidepressant treatment for the third group, who then did well. And those in the fourth group are going to need our support for a long time, while the real source of the problem(s) is gradually and therapeutically discovered.

It all made such sense, and, as I thought over my current caseload at the time, I could easily define who seemed to fit into which category. My biggest problem, as yours may be, was to find a way to help Group 2, without discouraging them to the point where they became even more dysfunctional.

I found that a useful device, for all four categories, was to study the dissociative disorders comparative chart with them, pointing out where they probably fit in and explaining the concepts. The negative self-hypnosis was one of the most important aspects to study and explain, along with very direct suggestion regarding self-talk. This is particularly important with Groups 2 and 4, as you can appreciate. I became quite dictatorial at times, insisting on "homework"; and, if I thought that they would disregard the instructions to say a positive sort of mantra ten times every day, I would make them write it out and bring it in. Writing it out is a type of self-hypnosis in itself, and it is important to make their posthypnotic suggestions in the positive, rather than the conditional, mode. When they have it written, there in front of them (and you), you can both look at the way the suggestion is described, literally at the words that the patient used, and modify them appropriately. ("Hmmm. Do you think that that's the best way to describe how you're feeling?" "Maybe you have another word in mind now that you look at it again." "Whoops! We've got a negative there—let's put it into the positive mode.")

Rather than the popular "Every day in every way I'm getting better and better", which is too open, or "if I get better I can …", it is important to rephrase it: "It is wonderful to be well again!"

51

My definition of an affirmation has this important proviso: it is in the positive mode, and it is very specific. The subconscious, always on the alert for danger, seems to disregard provisionary self-talk. Therefore it is a statement about the future, made in the present tense, as if it had already happened in the past. The blurred timelines ensure a hypnotic response. Hence my approval of "It is wonderful to be well again!"

You may choose to take the opportunity to discuss the role of early family life, pointing out that what may be unimportant in some families (because there are, among other things, enough positives to take up the slack) may seem insurmountable in others. Sometimes the insurmountable can be coped with only by burying it. However, when we bury emotions they have a nasty way of reincarnating themselves when we least expect them and are least able to cope with them. As with any dissociative disorders, a gentle "Tell me what it was like when you were growing up" offers a reasonably neutral invitation. You'll surely have a sense of how secure the attachment process was, and whether the child felt safe and/or had a safe person to go to when things got tough.

Somewhat related to this, there was an extremely interesting study done with patients who had a twin who was *not* affected with chronic fatigue syndrome. Basically the study set out to explore comorbid conditions, looking for relationships between the ten most common clinical conditions associated with significant fatigue: fibromyalgia, irritable bowel syndrome, multiple chemical sensitivities, temporomandibular joint disorder, interstitial cystitis, postconcussion syndrome, tension headache, chronic low back pain, chronic pelvic pain in women, and chronic nonbacterial prostatitis. The researchers felt that it was crucial to adjust for the effects of psychiatric illness, which can and does skew the presentations of such chronic disorders. Having made those comparisons, they then compared the patients with their nonfatigued twins. They found that the presence of comorbidity was definitely higher in the fatigued twin, and stated that comorbid states must always be considered if we are to give comprehensive treatment. I would add that, if your patient has a twin who does not seem to have the same crushing disorders, it would be interesting to ask the twin what it was like for him or her, during the childhood years. We all know that siblings often describe their growing-up years entirely differently; with suffering and nonsuffering twins, it would be even more interesting.

Another twin study (Sabath et al., 2002) showed differences in some cellular immunity factors, and, of course, immunological deficiencies have long been thought of as being part of the CFS vulnerability. This study is unique because the genetic factors are so much better controlled. Significantly greater variability, the study reports, was found in twins where one was affected by CFS and the other not.

Natelson and Lange (2002) still refer to CFS as being a medically unexplained condition, which may include rheumatological symptoms, signs of infectious agents (at least at the onset), and neuropsychiatric symptoms. It is thought, according to these authors, that no convincing data exist that explain continuance of infectious factors as the disease goes on (and on, and on).

Several other articles and reports are described in Chapter Seventeen.

I'm fairly sure that, in the ensuing decades, different names will be found for what we now call CFS. Whatever they may be, the patient will be in the same sorts of situation as today's patients are. Let us hope that medical science continues to explore, and offers even better explanations and solutions.

Somatization

There is an interesting boundary between somatization disorder and somatoform dissociation. One—the former—does seem to have an element of secondary gain, which is absent, or at least minimal, in the latter.

Neither, however, can be classified as "malingering". These are not symptoms that are intentionally invented to deceive. They are the desperate screams from the psyche by way of the body, that shout, "I am not well! Help!"

Mrs. D. was so desperate for help that she even agreed to come into my office. This was a huge effort for her, because she knew that germs lurked everywhere in doctors' offices. The fact that my office, by this time, was for psychotherapy and clinical hypnosis, and not a medical clinic, did nothing to ease her distress.

She would come in with her own sheet, which she would drape carefully over my very comfortable reclining chair, being sure to tuck it in beneath each arm, behind the headrest, along the side of the seat itself. The whole effort took several minutes. She brought her own towel, too, in case her hands got sweaty. I offered paper towels and/or tissues but those came from boxes and the boxes had been who-knows-where. When she got up to leave, she would very carefully stow the sheet in a plastic bag, turned and folded so as not to contaminate herself, in order to carry it home. I assume she dumped it directly into strong disinfectant when she got there.

She had specifically asked for some hypnosis, but her tense body pretty well sabotaged any such effort. There was no question in my mind that she was desperate, but I didn't really know how to help her. In the end, after three excruciating sessions, she chose not to return and so I felt that I hadn't really helped her at all.

There have been many other patients, equally compulsive in their own way. The message is one of terror, I finally decided—but terror of what, they could not say. *Something is dreadfully wrong. Find it and cure me, please, please.* But, as soon as one set of symptoms have abated, others are quick to take their place. Being well seems to be equated with being ill.

If you will look at the charts again on Pages 43 and 44, you will see the overlapping symptoms. Again, the negative self-hypnosis and the helpless/hopeless syndrome are prominent. Also of note is the distortion of body image. Sleep disturbances, nightmares and various other psychological diagnoses are similar to those we find in the dissociative spectrum. However, sleep deprivation, as opposed to disturbance, is not a very large factor; it is in PTSD, but not in DDNOS or DID and not in somatization disorder.

Working with somatization patients is a challenge. I think the countertransference is one of our biggest problems. We long to say, or shout, "There's nothing physically wrong with you! Just get on with your life!"

But they can't.

One of my ploys is to cajole them into finding one, just one, part of their bodies that they like. It may even be a toenail or their ears, it doesn't matter what it is. With that one little thing that they perhaps might grudgingly admit they like about themselves, the prison wall has a tiny crack in it.

If you think that all of this is becoming reminiscent of Chapter One and the thick-chart patient, of course you are right: it is. However, a major difference lies in the reason for the thick chart. Is it a somatization situation, or have we different ego states making their statements here? Once again, the line between chronic disorders and dissociative disorders is very thin.

These days, I do give somatization patients various diagnostic questionnaires for dissociation, if they will agree to do them. If the results seem to indicate a significant degree of dissociativity, then the line between ego-state representation and somatoform dissociation must be clarified. If the dissociation scales do *not* indicate a dissociative disorder, then the probability is that we have somatization disorder. Nevertheless, you can under-stand the commonalities and help your patient to understand them, too.

Some depressions

We need to differentiate between a depressed ego state, which can be found in every dissociative patient, and depression as the pri-mary diagnosis. This is best accomplished by simply observing the other phenomenology. Usually, the varying presentations of different ego states make the differentiation for us.

I am not talking here about reactive depressions, or those due to some other disease such as hypothyroidism, or those found in some alcoholics. Rather, these depressions seem to have "no reason" for being there. The lifestyle seems adequate, family life appears to be supportive. Why, then, the depression? Nobody knows. It seems to be endogenous. The situation may or may not respond to medication but this is one instance where I do feel that an adequate trial of an SSRI, such as paroxetine, is indicated. (As I mentioned previously, I also feel it is indicated when the depressed ego state is so very afflicted that it contaminates the whole system and no therapeutic work can be done until the black cloud is lifted.)

Distortions in cognitive thought play a major, and very negative, role here. The negative self-hypnosis is relentless and, of course, reinforces and exacerbates with every utterance. Furthermore, there tends to be right cerebral lateralization, also found in DDNOS and DID. There might be nightmares. Cognitive, cognitive/behavioral and dialectical/behavioral approaches are useful. They are best utilized, I find, by those who have specific training, especially the dialectical/behavioral techniques. As family physicians, we are well able to treat mild and even moderate depressions; however, men and women with these deep soul-searing depressions usually need more help than the family doc can give; it's time for the troops to call in the reinforcements. This also applies to those pathological grief reactions that seem to just take on a life of their own. Even the patient him- or herself often states, "I just don't know why I can't get over this—he died seven years ago. It's ridiculous that I can't get over it—" and then dissolves into buckets of tears again. Of all the various depressions, I consider these horrendous engulfments by grief, unrelenting even after many years, to be the most highly dissociative.

I must make one thing very clear. The comparative charts to which I have been referring come from my own interpretations of the many papers and presentations I have read, heard, and studied, along with my own personal experience. So, when you see four plus signs (++++), it is my impressions that you are seeing, not specific numbers. Where you see blanks or question marks, it is because I have not found sufficient evidence and/or references in the literature to hazard a guess. Take the comparative charts, then, as useful guidelines (which I believe they are) and never as written-in-stone fact.

What can you do?

With each of the topics discussed in this chapter, I do suggest exploring the similarities (and differences, of course!) with the dissociative disorders and getting a sense of whether the patient finds the comparisons interesting and/or useful. Naturally, you will be careful about how the dissociative aspect is described and a clear differentiation between the patient's problems and a dissociative disorder will be established.

Having done that, see what you might feel comfortable doing with the ego-state approaches. These really do bring the patient into the therapeutic arena and most patients appreciate it. If you are trained in clinical hypnosis, that too can be very helpful when you choose patient and diagnosis carefully.

Use the diagnostic questionnaires for dissociative disorders, especially the DES, DDIS (or SCID-D, but it's so long), and SDQ-20, to clarify dissociative status. I think the SDQ-20 is essential in all disorders where there is an overtone of somatization, to differentiate from somatoform dissociation.

Work on your countertransference!

To reiterate:

- as in the previous chapter, the disorders described here all have significant overlapping with various dissociative phenomena
- discussing these similarities with the patient can be helpful in some cases
- remember the differences between somatization and malingering

- clarify whether the situation seems to be somatoform dissociation or not
- call for help from psychological colleagues trained in other techniques when it is appropriate, such as with deep depressions.

Chapter Seven
Other Organ Systems

Irritable bowel syndrome

If ulcerative colitis expresses the essence of the phrase "gut reaction", irritable bowel syndrome (IBS) expresses it in spades.

As is the case with the topics described earlier, IBS seems to have "no cause". Of course, there must be a cause; we just aren't smart enough to have found it yet. What we do know is that it makes life miserable for thousands of people around the world. It also seems to be somewhat limited to the Western industrialized world, but I always wonder what the other cultures and countries have instead. Maybe it is a matter of definition.

IBS is frequently thought to be a disorder of bowel motility, although not all authors and researchers agree. It is almost surely unconnected to any infectious agents; as far as I know, it does not carry any increased risk for malignancies, as is sometimes thought to be the case with ulcerative colitis. Among many excellent review articles, an older contribution by Lynn and Friedman (1995) is certainly worth reading. They comment on the frequent assumption that IBS is caused by altered colonic motility, especially, it seems, in the ascending colon. However, Farthing (1995) summed it up very succinctly when he wrote, "Debate continues on whether the irritable bowel syndrome is a condition in which abnormal motility is normally perceived or in which normal motility is abnormally perceived" (page 172).

Another of my favorite articles is that of Goldberg and Davidson (1997). They have titled it "A biopsychosocial understanding of the irritable bowel syndrome: a review".

Almost all articles refer to comorbid factors, especially psychosocial problems. Several writers refer to the predominance of a history of childhood physical or sexual abuse (Drossman and

Thompson, 1992; Thompson, 1994; Talley, 2002). Understanding my predilection for seeing dissociation hiding behind every psychosocial tree, you will no doubt understand my interpretation of IBS as *also* having dissociative characteristics. Some authors have described this as being "learned-illness behavior" (which sounds a lot like "blame the patient") but then, almost all dissociative characteristics could be so classified, as the responses were learned coping skills that the child developed in order to manage the world.

IBS seems to affect an astonishing percentage of the population; estimates of 10 to 20 percent are common in North America, the United Kingdom, and The Netherlands. That being the case, one wonders why it still seems to be such a mystery disease. More latterly, emphasis has been put on psychosocial factors and therefore on stress management, relaxation techniques, hypnosis, group therapy and cognitive behavioral approaches. An article in *The Medical Post* on 10 August 1995 tells of new pharmaceutical interventions that look promising. However, I wonder whether this is again going to be a situation wherein the medication is helpful in controlling symptoms, but does nothing toward relieving the underlying causes.

And then we must, as always, consider our own reactions to patients with IBS. Van Dulmen et al. (1994) addressed the situation. They stated, "Doctors have to perceive patients' cognitions and emotions in order to change them" (page 582), and then went on to describe the differences, which their study brought to light, in doctors' perceptions, underestimations and overestimations. They commented that doctors had to learn which questions to ask; then they went on to state that it wasn't enough just to know what to look for (and ask about)—we also need to have the skills to discern what they call "patients' complaint-related cognitions and behavior". It is an article well worth reading.

And it brings me back to the dissociative aspect of all chronic disorders, including IBS.

The link that several authors make, to early childhood trauma, certainly highlights the possibility of dissociative response. However, it recapitulates, once again, this question: is this somatoform dissociation, or a form of somatization precipitated many years ago by abuse?

Does it really matter? you might wisely ask.

Yes, because, once again, if it is basically somatoform dissociation we must begin to think in terms of a significant dissociative element in that patient's life and start exploring this. Referral for evaluation to a therapist knowledgeable in dissociative disorders may be appropriate. On the other hand, somatization—which can be and often is precipitated by trauma—is a different kettle of fish and, although that patient, too, may benefit from an ego-state approach, it is not with the same underlying psychopathology.

What can you do?

Let's focus on the IBS patient in whom you do not suspect an underlying major dissociative disorder.

First, find out what the patient herself wants, besides having the whole thing disappear. Does she want information about the newest medications? Does she want better coping skills? What might the patient already be doing with regard to stress management and how knowledgeable is she about the links between stress and physiological response—the mind–body connection? These are always good places to start, and there are almost always stress-management groups around somewhere, where relaxation, self-hypnosis and other self-calming techniques are taught.

Explore the possibility that the patient might make friends with her digestive system. It may sound bizarre, but then the outrageous often works where sound reason doesn't. Such an approach might include dialogues between patient and bowel, or learning to focus on the intestinal tract in a positive rather than a negative way. After all, there must be some degree of good function, or the person would be more physically ill. Self-hypnosis using imagery of comfortable and healthy digestive-system functioning can be very useful. The same goes for learning a positive vocabulary, such as "my bowel is moving in comfortable, healthy wavelike patterns".

As a doctor, check out your own perceptions of the patient's experience, and her perception of *your* understanding of that experience. In order to do that, be aware of what authors describe as "Abnormal illness attitudes in patients with irritable bowel syndrome", which is the title of an article by Gomborone et al. (1995). In it there is a very interesting graph ("Illness Attitude Scale") that compares IBS with normal volunteers, patients with organic disease and patients who are depressed. They point out that both the IBS group and the depressed group show higher scores than the organic group in three areas: effects of symptoms on the person's feelings and emotions; worry about illness; and death phobia. They also point out that the IBS group scored higher than any of the other groups on hypochondriacal beliefs, what they term "disease phobia", and bodily preoccupation.

And then, while you are contemplating these graphs and implications, remember that we must always include our own attitudes about how patients "should" feel and what they "should" understand. As many authors point out (including yours truly), a strong therapeutic alliance is vital in any ongoing relationship with a patient who has a debilitating illness, and much more so when that illness has strong mind-body aspects that are constantly interacting. The basis of such a therapeutic alliance is healthy respect for what each other is describing.

I must make reference to a veteran in the field of IBS and the use of hypnosis to alleviate symptoms, P. J. Whorwell (Houghton, Heyman, and Whorwell, 1996). He has authored and/or co-authored two seminal papers, many years ago when it was not common to suggest that physicians consider such far-out approaches as clinical hypnosis for "medical problems". My guess—a fairly educated one, I think—is that success for hypnosis in this area depends as much on the beliefs of the therapist who does the hypnosis, and the physician who may have referred the patient, as it does on the attitudes of the patient herself. Whorwell believed, and inspired his patients to do the same, and he found significant improvement.

Urinary problems

After all appropriate investigations have been carried out, chronic urinary disorders that do not seem to have "any cause" may reasonably be explored from a trauma-history perspective.

It doesn't take a great leap of understanding to make the connection between GU problems and a history of sexual abuse. There are some internationally acclaimed authors and researchers in the field who have published reams about this—van der Kolk, van der Hart, Steele, Nijenhuis, to name only a few.

We must be very careful about several aspects of such situations:

- Avoiding implying that the problem is "all in your mind". This tops the list.
- Dismissing the problem as unimportant because it *is* psychosomatic.
- Too quick a referral to a psychiatrist or psychologist. Patients do better when we take the time to explain the mind–body connection, implicit versus explicit memory, and how we all have resources within ourselves that can be accessed when we are taught how to do that.
- Reassuring the patients that we will go on this journey *with* them, not "dump" them.
- Suggesting reading material for them. Our patients are not intellectually challenged; they can read as well as we can. The reading material can open the gate to discussing the mind–body aspects together, which is always a very positive thing to do, for both parties; it really establishes and improves the therapeutic alliance that some of us are always bleating about.
- Helping the patient to feel that we really do understand that they are suffering and we are looking for all possible ways to relieve that suffering.

Many family physicians can undertake such discussions themselves, either before making the referral or as an adjunct to it. Some are able to do the counseling themselves, too, but that can lead to a confusion of roles, which ultimately may not be helpful.

Every case is different in these regards. Besides, some patients may need more than counseling—good psychotherapy may be in order.

In some situations, physical scarring from early sexual abuse may be a major contributing factor to the urinary distress (horrible thought, but true). Such scarring should have been identified in the "appropriate investigations" to which I referred at the beginning of this section. This may lead to long discussions about the relative merits of plastic surgery, should the scarring be causing irritation and/or interfering with urinary tract function.

Many physicians are amazed, if this path is taken, to find that the patients have never told anybody about the abuse before. (This is contrary to some allegations that patients are keen on making up stories of abuse. Very few do. Most are so ashamed of it that they never have told anybody. Can you imagine what it is like to be ashamed of the fact that one or some adults did very, very nasty things to you when you were a child?)

This indicates to us how important it is to include appropriate and sensitive questioning about abuse issues, especially when the symptoms are not corroborated by functional, anatomical and/or physiological aspects. Even when scarring is present, those questions may never have been asked. Ask them.

There may also be real pathology, such as persistent or chronic infections, that are related to the scarring. Furthermore, such infections may be a result of the patients' repeated scrubbing of the urogenital areas in a desperate endeavor to keep themselves clean—equating past abuse with physical or moral uncleanness. In turn, these misinterpretations may have been traumatically invoked and stored in their implicit memory banks and barely recognized as cognitive but inappropriate behaviors.

Anything having to do with problems "down there" is difficult for many people to speak about, even in order to seek advice from their family physician. Careful history taking is again the key to good physical and emotional healthcare.

Another aspect of urogenital problems may be promiscuity by an ego state whose role is focused on sexuality. Other parts of the personality structure may not even know about this behavior and will very likely be appalled if and when they are told about it. This is a case where good communication with the patient's psychotherapist is extremely important. He or she needs to know about repeated sexually transmitted diseases, for example. Testing for the more dangerous STD's should be delicately handled. A signed release of information is always a good thing to have and should go both ways—physician to therapist and therapist to physician. You can understand how important it is to have a frank and open discussion with the patients, who are often prone to consider such sharing as a breach of trust.

Neurological anomalies

Pseudoseizures are among the many neurological disturbances that can occur with trauma-spectrum disorders.

The diagnostic investigations are complicated by the fact that many trauma survivors do have EEG abnormalities—especially in the temporal lobes—that are not transformed into seizure behavior; so, on the one hand, we have EEG indications of seizure activity, which the patient doesn't experience, and on the other we have apparent seizures, but there are no EEG changes. Life is never simple.

Dr. Elizabeth Bowman wrote about the phenomenon of pseudoseizures, comparing occurrence with real seizures in dissociative patients, long before anybody else was paying much attention. She found, in one early study (Bowman, 1993) that 88 percent of the subjects had sustained significant trauma, including both physical and sexual abuse. When looking for the most common psychodynamic pathways, she and her colleagues ascertained that, most commonly, dissociated ego states were expressing memories of abuse, and that these memories had been triggered by recent stressors or traumatic events.

In an article with the wonderful title "Pseudoseizures, Families and Unspeakable Dilemmas", Griffith et al. (1998) confirmed that in thirteen of fourteen family interviews an unspeakable dilemma was evident, and also that the identified patient was the most silent member of the family. The authors pointed out the importance of family therapy.

More recently, Salmon et al. (2003) corroborated that, in non-epileptic seizures, only child psychological abuse uniquely distinguished them from epileptic seizures. Furthermore, this link virtually always had to do with family dysfunction.

As family physicians, then, we obviously need to keep these highly possible origins in mind when dealing with apparent seizure activity, but negative neurological findings to explain it.

Pseudocomatose states

"Marlene," my friend Erica said to me one day when I was visiting, "can I talk to you about Joanna?" She was referring to another friend who had been staying with her a few weeks previously. I had met Joanna on several occasions, and liked her, and I knew that the two of them had been friends for many years.

"Of course," I replied.

What she then went on to describe was a situation that had happened some time before, when Joanna had also been staying with Erica. Apparently, Joanna had been becoming more and more withdrawn, saying little and apparently being very introspective; then one day she had simply taken to her bed. She was breathing regularly, had a good pulse and color, but could not be awakened yet didn't seem to be asleep, either.

"It was like she was in a coma," Erica said. The doctor had been called, and came; he found nothing specific and suggested overwhelming fatigue.

Joanna ate nothing—at least, as far as anyone could tell—and no one even saw her go to the bathroom. "But she must have," Erica said, "because it would be impossible to go for six days without emptying your bladder, even if you're not drinking, wouldn't it?"

I agreed. "Maybe she gets up in the middle of the night, when you're asleep," I suggested.

Maybe," Erica agreed. "But, you know, Joanna had a terrible childhood. She had a vicious mother and an alcoholic father. You and I have talked about your work with dissociation, so I'm wondering—do you think this "coma" stuff could be dissociation rather than real coma? That she *wouldn't*, rather than couldn't, be aroused?"

I hadn't seen a case of pseudocoma before, but it made sense. Apparently, Joanna had risen from her bed after six days, as if nothing had happened. She didn't talk about the situation, just passed it off with a shrug. It was almost as if she had been in a self-imposed fugue state, from the way Erica described it.

A couple of years later, both Joanna and I happened to be staying with Erica at the same time. For some reason, we started to talk about sleep habits; I commented to Joanna that she seemed to sleep like the dead (she didn't even stir when I went past her to get to the bathroom to have a shower) and she agreed. "Oh, yes," she replied, "I've always been like that. Sometimes people get worried about me. But it's just me—I'm fine." And she changed the subject.

The more I thought about it, the more I came to the conclusion that these were pseudocomatose states that Joanna went into when being with people became too difficult. I don't even think they were deliberate, that is, not cognitively decided. They just happened. They were a form of protection, originating in that good old protective subconscious. Because she was staying with other people, she needed a way to absent herself for a period of time, perhaps days, in order to be "with" everybody again. So she fell into this strange sort of "coma". The fact that it upset others didn't seem to register with her.

Not much has been written about pseudocoma. When one does find an article or two, it seems always to be considered as a conversion disorder. So far, the most relevant piece I have found on conversion disorders is by Dr. Mark Landau (2001). The article deals with many sets of symptoms that affect voluntary motor or sensory function, including pseudocoma and pseudoseizures. To him, conversion disorders represent a type of somatoform disorder, and he very clearly differentiates them from factitious disorders and malingering. He makes a point that conversion symptoms are not under intentional or voluntary control, and states, "Patients with conversion disorders may present with hemiparesis, paraparesis, monoparesis, alteration of conscious-ness, visual loss, eizurellike [seizure-like] activity, pesudocoma, abnormal gait disturbance, aphonia, lack of coordination, or a bizarre movement disorder." I was cheered to find, under his differential diagnosis, "dissociative disorders".

Personally, I don't much care for the term "conversion disorder", which does have an aroma of intentionality about it, despite Landau's disclaimer. I do agree, however, that this may well be a type of somatoform dissociation and, as such, would warrant a little exploration into the possibility of an underlying dissociative disorder—even something as mild as "tell me what it was like when you were growing up".

Sensory aberrations

These are not all that rare with dissociative conditions, and may be relegated either to one or two ego states, or pervade much of the system. They are often described as tingling and/or numb-ness along some part of the body. Neurological testing, in the form of electrical conduction studies or evoked potentials, is usually normal. (These sorts of situation are where a lot of psychiatrist-versus-neurologist dilemmas surface.) As always, in good medical practice, the symptoms deserve investigation, but not twenty times over. Once, with perhaps one second opinion if the patient is very worried, should be enough. A trauma history is important for the investigation specialist to know about; naturally it is kept in perspective. There are all too many situations where a superficial investigation of a patient predetermined to be "neurotic" has failed to elicit the proper diagnosis; that must be avoided at all costs. In other words, this is again like walking the tightrope. Keep the balance bar firmly in hand.

Usually it evolves that the sensory abnormality is there to serve some purpose within the system. In other words, it is a safety net. It may keep the patient going to doctors (with ongoing visits to specialists) or quite the opposite—prevent the patient from talking about something because, if she talks about it, the sensory discomfort increases.

One of my dearest patients had had a grisly childhood, being transferred from one foster home to another for many years. As part of her abuse, she remembers being covered by snakes and consequently almost always was plagued with the sensation of snakes all over her. We worked long and hard on that sensation and in time I was permitted to meet the ego state who was "the Keeper of the Snakes". Eventually, we all reached a compromise wherein the keeper of the snakes would watch me closely and, if I was doing something she considered dangerous, she would let me know.

Therapy went along blissfully for several months. Then, one day, the patient came in, white as a sheet and shaking.

"What on earth has happened?"

"The snakes are back."

I asked to speak to the Keeper of the Snakes and, to my relief, she emerged. "Help me to understand this," I asked.

"She was *talking too much, of course!*"

Of course. When as a child, she tried to tell people what was happening to her, she was punished more, and so talking to me about her abuse put her in the same precarious position and the Keeper of the Snakes was, in that upside-down way one finds so often when working with dissociation, determined to protect her.

Hence the miserable sensory experience of snakes crawling all over her.

You will probably not be in the position of therapist and so will not have to play the same role in working through the causative factors, but it is helpful to know that this sort of thing can happen.

Numbness or tingling is the more common presentation. I usually ask what the symptoms prevent the patient from doing, which often gives some clue as to which ego state might be playing a role. Very often, though, it doesn't prevent the patient from doing anything, it is just "there".

Non-anatomical pain patterns

Almost all dissociative patients have one or more ego states whose job it is to experience the pain. This means that other parts of the system do not have to experience pain. Very often it is a child part (which seems, on the face of it, to be particularly unfair).

This needs to be kept in mind when the patient has to go in the hospital for some reason, such as a fracture that needs to be reduced, or any other situation where pain is an expected result; it is not uncommon to find such patients walking around the corridors when they should still be resting the affected part of their anatomy. "But it doesn't hurt *at all* and I'm so *bored*," she might wail.

No, it doesn't hurt at all, because that other ego state is experiencing it all for her. You'll need to make your orders very clear to that patient, and to the nursing staff. Usually, if you and the patient have developed sufficient rapport and she knows that you understand the dissociation, you can just be upfront about the situation.

On the other hand, it might be one part of the body that is in excruciating pain for no apparent reason and with no known anatomical rationale, such as, "My whole left side, right from the top of my head, is in terrible pain." Another patient of mine, a professional woman, has to take to her bed because of the whole-body pain that often consumes her, especially after a difficult situation with a colleague. I am trusting that, as we continue to work through all her past trauma, the pain will abate. She doesn't share my optimism.

As you might expect, medication is usually completely ineffective with this type of pain. Something like a tricyclic antidepressant might work in very small doses. Stay away from the big guns—morphine, other opiates, haloperidol, etc.

Usually I focus on stress management and relaxation techniques. If you can link up an exacerbation of pain with a difficult time in therapy, this is usually accepted by the patient. Ask if it is all right for you to discuss it with her therapist.

This chapter is a mere cross-section of some of the more common, apparently bizarre expressions of trauma-spectrum disorders. You will find more information about relevant psychoneurophysiology in Chapters Seventeen and Nineteen.

To reiterate:

- people who have had trauma in their lives, especially in childhood, often have physiological responses that relate to the trauma
- irritable bowel syndrome is often considered to be somatoform in nature
- chronic urinary tract and urogenital problems may be related to trauma
- strange neurophysiological presentations, such as pseudo-seizures, are usually reflective of a psychological need
- all symptoms are real to the patient, and all deserve our professional attention.

Chapter Eight
Post-traumatic Stress Disorder Symptoms

Ed was a 52-year-old man who had served not one but three stints in Vietnam. When it seemed as if he was about to be sent off again, he "borrowed" a jeep and drove to Canada. (He has since received amnesty.)

His presenting complaint was of marital problems. Although it seemed that he and his wife truly cared for each other, she was ready to leave. They had a little girl, just three years old, whom they both adored, and Ed was desperate to find some solution that would save not only the relationship with his wife, but the family unit itself.

He was the first to admit that he was difficult to live with, and that this was the third relationship to go on the rocks, although neither of the previous two had been as important to him as this one. He also recognized, very clearly, that he was "difficult to live with" and that the problem was based, in large measure, on his Vietnam experiences. Intellectually, he knew all about it—the lack of ability to trust, the hypervigilance, the flashbacks, the "surliness" that was his depression getting deeper and deeper. What he didn't know was how to get well. He belonged to a group of Vietnam veterans who got together semimonthly to encourage each other, and that helped, but not nearly enough.

Originally, he came into my office because I ran a group for people who wanted (they all said) to stop smoking. Actually, they all wanted to be nonsmokers but they did not want to stop smoking—an uncomfortable reality that they had, reluctantly, to face.

During one session, I asked his intellectual, grown-up part to reassure his teenage "smoking is a cool thing to do" part that it was OK now to stop smoking. To the astonishment of everyone in the group, including me, he burst out, "No! No! It's not OK! I know, when I'm smoking, that I'm safe!" As it eventually turned out, they were allowed to smoke only back at the base, never when they were on patrol because the sight or smell of the smoke might alert the enemy. So he was right—smoking represented safety. But the outburst was typical PTSD: for those few moments, he was back in the jungle.

After the final session he came up to me and asked if I knew anyone who worked with PTSD. He already knew that I worked with people who had PTSD, but this was just his way of initiating an uncomfortable query. We clarified that I did indeed know something about such things, and he became a patient. He was dedicated, gritted his teeth to get through some of the sessions, worked hard, did his "homework", and suffered. They all suffer, terribly.

In a way, all dissociative disorders could be called "post-traumatic stress disorders". One would simply have to differentiate between those cases arising from childhood trauma and those arising from other kinds of trauma such as war, rape, accident, stalking, floods, being caught in an avalanche, or the myriad other disasters that could, and do, leave a lasting imprint on the mind and body—an emotional scar on the psyche.

We know that those who are most vulnerable, those who are most at risk of developing PTSD should they be caught up in other catastrophic circumstances later in life, are those who have had that notorious "dysfunctional childhood". That was shown clearly in all the research done on the veterans from the Vietnam War. Those soldiers were not necessarily dissociative at the time of joining the military forces and being sent overseas, but their experiences early in life were disruptive, emotionally or physically painful, confusing, or some combination of such vulnerabilities. This is common to virtually all people with post-traumatic stress symptoms. It is as if the brain has been sensitized by the previous experiences, and is then unable to respond in any way other than traumatically, connecting and registering within the limbic memory banks the overwhelming disproportionate response of PTSD. It is neither intentional nor cognitive, and therefore almost impossible for the patient to understand, prevent, stop, or correct.

Neurophysiology and neurochemistry

These factors will be discussed in much greater detail in Chapters Sixteen and Nineteen.

Severe stress, occurring over prolonged periods of time, or that which is overwhelming in its intensity even during a shorter period of time, changes the biochemistry of the brain and the body. Until a very short time ago, it was thought that these changes—particularly to the biochemistry—were forever. Now it seems that this may not be the case: with the advent of the new theories of neurogenesis, it is perhaps possible that neurological repair can indeed be achieved. We don't really know enough about that yet, but intense research is going on. However, we do know that people who suffer severe PTSD, dating back many decades, still have recognizable and measurable neurochemical changes and presumably neurophysiology is similarly affected.

Because the very basis of neurophysiological response is compromised, it is unrealistic to expect fast results, a return to "normality" in people who have been severely traumatized. Rather, it is a long-term return to what we think of as normality; in many cases, however, it has to do with learning new coping skills rather than the usual definition of what constitutes healing, which we think of as once again being what one was before, in terms of self-worth, good personal skills, and achievement goals.

PTSD is a complex issue, so it is the more common aspects and presenting symptoms that will be discussed in the following pages.

Panic attacks

Among the most common problems related to PTSD that are encountered in general practice are panic attacks. Of course, this is not to say that all panic attacks have PTSD at their source, but it is there to some degree in a remarkable percentage of such cases.

A panic attack is a wonderful example of the neurophysiology of trauma. Some trigger, something ordinarily thought of as innocuous, instantaneously links up with an implicit memory in the prefrontal cortex and the whole adrenergic system explodes.

We are all familiar with the old fight-or-flight response. In fact, it is now recognized that there is a third aspect to that response, which actually comes first: freeze! (see Figure 16.1: Stress and the brain on page 139).

Observation of any animal—or, for that matter, small child—that is suddenly faced with an unexpected and potentially dangerous situation, will clearly show the first reaction, which is to freeze. It may only last a few seconds, but it is there. *Then* comes fight or flight. But what do you do when you can neither fight nor flee? Somehow one has to do something, so the good old adrenals respond to the immediate spurt of hypothalamic-pituitary action and send out their emergency response team—the hormonal outpouring that gives our bodies immediate weaponry: increased heartbeat, respiratory change, blood flow directed to the musculature, all of which are required for action. But there's nothing to act *on*, no visible danger, no one to talk to or even yell at, nothing. So what does the body do? It goes into panic-attack mode, of course. All those hormones running around have to be used up somehow. And the person is overcome with the intense fear that accompanies panic, when there is no way to escape.

Sometimes just explaining the response, the way I have explained it above, will help the person cope with the attacks. More often, though, some simple techniques such as controlled breathing, a little self-hypnosis and/or posthypnotic suggestion, code words, and the like, are needed. It means taking time with the patients to work with them, and it is time very well spent, both for the patient and for the physician, who almost surely will otherwise receive many more calls in the middle of the night, from patients or their frantic relatives, or from the emergency department of the local hospital.

Medication is sometimes required. Both anxiolytics and small doses of SSRI antidepressants such as paroxetine, which boost the serotonergic system, can be helpful. However, I am (as you may have already discerned) a notorious non-pill-giver, and prefer working with the alternatives first. If such techniques can be helpful, they prevent adverse responses and/or sensitization to pharmaceuticals, and they also empower the patient, which is surely a huge advantage however one looks at it.

Above all, reassure the patient that he is not crazy and, further-more, will not go crazy. It is just that super-protective subconscious, doing its best to take care of the person in the best way it knows how—by getting the mind–body connection working as quickly as possible. As with many kinds of misery, the road toward it is paved with best (subconscious) intentions.

Hypervigilance

Hypervigilance is another of the very disruptive PTSD symptoms. It drives to distraction not only the patient involved, but his friends and family even more so. Many a spousal or family quarrel has erupted because Mom or Dad, brother or sister, has shouted out, "For heaven's sake! There's nothing there! What are you so uptight about?" Of course, the language may be a little more colorful than what I have just used. Frequently, it will be a family member who comes into the doctor's office for help, perhaps disguised with a symptom of his or her own, such as anxiety or depression or loss of anger control. (As a side note, this is one of the huge advantages that a family physician has, as we all know: because we are connected to the family, not just a solitary patient, we have a better immediate understanding of where the source of a problem may lie.)

Hypervigilance—the intense need to always, always be on the lookout for danger, whether there is any obvious source or not—is one of the most common indications of a post-traumatic stress disorder. It is, again, a response at the level of the subconscious mind, probably originating in the orbitofrontal areas. That part of our brains is constantly scanning the horizon, as it were, in case something or someone presenting a potential threat is lurking there. The fact that there is almost never a potential threat lurking there is a conscious concept and makes no impact at all on the subconscious response.

It is not hard to understand. If one has been stalked, one is all too keenly aware of a shadow, a small sound, a possible footstep, an implicit message underlying the hanging up on the answering machine. The *fact*—for example, that the perpetrator is behind bars—holds no security.

Those who suffer from the worst kinds of hypervigilance will seldom go into a restaurant because they must, absolutely *must*, sit in a corner where nothing and nobody can get behind them. Similar responses severely limit social life and interrupt relationships, to say nothing of being very hard on the person himself, in a never-ending state of anxiety and "but-what-ifs".

There are some hypnotic techniques that can be helpful, although magic is hard to find these days. If you don't do hypnosis yourself (and that means having been properly trained by a fully professional hypnosis group) it is not hard to find a colleague who does. There are excellent training societies in virtually every country, certainly in the Western world, and the Asian countries have their own, very useful and appropriate, techniques.

At times, hypervigilance approaches paranoia, and it might be worth while discussing the situation with a psychiatrist or psychology colleague. This may be another of those situations where (horrors!) medication might be indicated, such as a very small dose of respiridone.

Hyperarousal

This is the physiological equivalent of hypervigilance. In a way, it is a specifically directed panic attack. Usually, however, the origin of the response is recognized, i.e. it doesn't so much come out of the blue, but develops from an escalating situation. It becomes a completely inappropriate response to what is perceived by others as a relatively minor situation. Knowing that doesn't help it to abate and in fact increases the agitation in the person having the symptoms.

As with panic attacks, it frequently leads to the emergency room and often to many otherwise unnecessary investigations. Never should disquieting symptoms that may indicate a heart attack, for example, be dismissed; but, when there has been good investigation done and all is normal, repeated investigations can be detrimental, especially emotionally. It is not uncommon, as we all know, for a suffering patient to demand, "Find out what's wrong!" I don't blame them. I would want to understand what's wrong, too. But what is wrong, after appropriate study has ruled out insidious causes, is found in the mind–body response and needs to be addressed from that perspective.

Once again, I would always start with a nonpharmaceutical technique such as mind–body communication work. It is better to empower the patient to control the situation whenever possible, before resorting to medication. Sometimes group work can be helpful. Just knowing that one is not alone in the world with these bizarre symptoms may lead the way to achieve self-regulation. It's hard work, though, which is also why group support is so very helpful.

Flashbacks

A flashback is not a memory. When we remember something, even if it was a terrible experience, we know where we are in time and space and that we are remembering a previous time. With a flashback, the person is right back in that time and space, and not in the present time at all. It is completely different.

All of the sensory stimuli are there: sight, sound, kinesthetic awareness, touch, smell—all of them. That is what makes it so terrifying. As with Ed and his outburst about knowing that he was safe when he could smoke, one is again completely present in that terrifying situation.

Often a flashback will occur at night, while one is sleeping, and the person may not know that it had happened, except that he wakes up drenched in sweat, with heart pounding and a sense of danger and doom. Sleep is, of course, disturbed, which is in itself a complicating factor. One's performance at work may be compromised; tempers are short; concentration is impaired.

People often ask, "When will the flashbacks go away?" Unfortunately, there is usually no easy answer for them. It is not like ordinary memory, even bad memories, which tend to fade as time passes. It is an entirely different mechanism that seems to persist even decades later. I think that most people eventually get relief when they have received good psychotherapy, as the old implicit, experiential memories are gradually processed through the hippocampus and become finally incorporated into the left brain's language-and-logic memory banks. Presumably, the subconscious triggers are then no longer so vulnerable, so easily aroused.

Nightmares

Nightmares are in a slightly different category. People awaken knowing that they have had a nightmare, also with heart pounding and a sense of fear. However, they appear to be recognized as nightmares, and therefore more easily understood. Even in sleep, there is apparently an awareness different from the sense of being back in the midst of the trauma. This is difficult to decipher, as people certainly perceive themselves to have "been there" in the nightmare, but perhaps the answer is that a flashback is recognizable as a real past experience that actually happened, whereas a nightmare is bizarre and not identified with reality.

Trust

As always with trauma, the victim loses the ability to trust. It is seen with all survivors of childhood trauma that has been inflicted by someone who was supposed to love and protect the child. Whom can you trust if you can't trust those whose very job is to love and protect you? It is unfair. Trusting becomes dangerous. It erodes the most basic of the attachment processes.

In a similar fashion, personal trauma that comes through no fault of one's own is also unfair and begins to erode one's trust in oneself, to say nothing of trusting the world around us. It becomes too difficult to put any faith in the world, or in people, because you had done that, and look what happened! And so being able to trust becomes virtually impossible. We can understand that some types of trauma fit into this explanation more readily than others: injury, emotional or physical or sexual, inflicted by another person or in other circumstances where we should have been able to trust our safety in those circumstances, will certainly erode trust very quickly. But, as I mentioned at the beginning of this chapter, those who have already had their attachments—their ability to trust—compromised when they were young are extremely susceptible to this process of emotional isolation. It plays havoc with all relationships, and especially with those in which trust is such an essential ingredient.

To refer again to the Vietnam veterans, the fact that they were degraded instead of met as heroes when they returned to the United States after the war added immeasurably to their agony. They had gone to serve their country. Those very people who should have lauded them instead derided them. It is no wonder that their trust—in this case, in their fellow Americans and in the government that sent them to war—was severely affected. It added to the injustice.

Many veterans of other wars have also suffered immeasurably from PTSD, but at least, in some of those conflicts, this particular component was not there. It is true, though, that PTSD has been misunderstood and misdiagnosed for a long time, and unspeakable things happened in other wars to soldiers whose terrible inner conflicts were totally disregarded and perceived in completely unjust ways—as cowards, for example. Many of them still will not talk about their war experiences; many of them still have debilitating symptoms. We may miss part of the diagnosis if we are not constantly aware of past experiences, even if those experiences happened decades ago.

Depression

Depression is often masked, and never more so than in someone with PTSD. It can underlie anger, which is quite common with this patient population. It is often expressed through physical symptoms, a sort of somatization. It may show up in sleep disturbances, or as fatigue. These attributes of depression are well known to us, and certainly not only found in people with PTSD, but bear remembering—especially the anger. It very often infects the whole personality, a sort of emotional virus, and psychological or psychiatric intervention may be necessary. It should never be ignored.

Often the patients will not, themselves, mention depression It's safer to always inquire, and particularly so when other aspects of PTSD are recognized. On the other hand, patients will come in with a presenting complaint of depression, which they have, but it is masking other PTSD symptoms. Usually in a family practice this will be recognized through our previous knowledge of the patient and his family. It is amazing, though, how many experiences our patients have had—about which we know almost nothing—that have been dismissed as passed and gone.

Other considerations

It is easy to make the connection with PTSD when the patient has been in combat, been assaulted, or suffered serious injury due to accident or some other phenomenon such as environmental disasters. However, we must remember two other factors.

First, it is not always in the forefront of our minds should the patient come in who has a near relative who has suffered those injuries. Vicarious traumatization is a real entity, and, more often than we realize, may be the root of distress in those who are close to the more easily perceived victim. Usually what presents is frustration—not hard to understand. But, underneath that, it is worthwhile to think of other PTSD factors: maybe a little counseling, or even just talking it out, is in order.

This vicarious suffering can be found in physicians and counselors, too. We need to take care of ourselves, and go to talk to someone if and when pressures become overwhelming.

Second, we always need to remember that emotional trauma is just as devastating as physical trauma, and PTSD from emotional battering is a real entity. This applies to bullying, belittling, and all the ways of undermining someone's sense of self. I have heard, and probably so have you, a patient say, "I just relive that situation, when he was yelling at me that way, for what seemed like hours—I think about it all the time and feel just like I'm back there again." This, also, is post-traumatic stress, even though we don't usually think of it in the same category as other kinds of disasters.

Third, in the DSM it states that "… in PTSD cognitive reality testing is intact", and of course that is usually true. However, that statement is *not* congruent with a flashback, in which the person is right back in the trauma and not in present reality at all.

An example came up recently for me what I was an expert witness in a court case. The Crown Prosecutor was determined to rely word for word on the DSM, and unwilling to see the obvious disjunction. Those of you who may find yourselves as a witness for the defense, Beware!

What can you do?

If possible, go to some courses on post-traumatic stress disorder, to learn a few techniques that can carry you through many of the office crises. Few of us are trained to be psychotherapists, but the basic techniques in handling immediate situations are not difficult to learn and there are some good workshops and conferences around. Such courses are interesting, and practical. Your new knowledge of the basic neurophysiology and neurobiochemical aspects will also be very useful. It also helps us to understand, and therefore have more empathy with, our patients.

I would also recommend very highly that you read the review, "The Body Keeps the Score" (van der Kolk, 1994).

Our patients recognize and appreciate our attempt to understand what it is like for them to be in this perpetual maelstrom of emotional and physiological response. Often, just that understanding and a willingness to listen—perhaps for the umpteenth time—is all that is needed in the moment. More specific work can come later.

Recognize when a referral to a psychiatrist or psychology colleague *who is known to work with trauma-spectrum disorders* is appropriate. In my part of the world, most psychiatrists tend to think of pharmaceutical remedies more quickly than do psychologists, but there are certainly times when medication is needed, and monitored. Remember, though, that patients may perceive referral as a way of being brushed off. Talk the situation over with them and explain your reason for referral, e.g. to ascertain whether medication would be helpful.

Perhaps you can organize a discussion group with colleagues, to meet once a month or so. Troublesome cases, which provoke exasperation and frustration in patient and doctor alike, can be discussed. If nothing else, there is comfort in company.

Take care of yourself. We can't be really helpful to others if we are not emotionally healthy ourselves.

To reiterate:

- post-traumatic stress disorder is a type of dissociative disorder
- it frequently presents as panic attacks, sleep disorders, or depression

- there are several well-recognized aspects that are almost always present: hypervigilance, hyperarousal, flashbacks, lack of trust
- in general, the treatment is psychotherapy
- the symptoms reflect a neurophysiological response that is persistent over long periods of time
- neurochemistry is changed in specific and identifiable ways
- referral to psychiatry or psychology colleagues may be indicated.

Chapter Nine
Comorbid States Associated with Dissociation

Depression

When we are considering and assessing possible comorbid states in patients who have a dissociative disorder, the question sometimes becomes, "Which diagnosis comes first?"

For example, virtually all people who are markedly dissociative, and are diagnosed with DID, will have a depressed ego state. During the time when that ego state is "out", the whole aspect of the patient is one of severe depression. At times, a severely depressed ego state will negatively affect the functioning of the whole system, and is one good reason for prescribing antidepressants, especially the SSRIs. Of course, one runs into the rebellion of other ego states who do not want to take the medication, but the answer there is fairly straightforward: "She needs it, she takes it; if you don't need it, you don't have to take it but the dose must be given to the body so that she can have it."

Depression is also commonly found in patients with DDNOS and those who suffer form PTSD. Once again, we must decide which is the primary diagnosis as far as we are concerned—the PTSD or the depression. This decision has a role in the way therapy is organized, and although this is primarily the purview of the therapist, it is the family physician who monitors the whole patient from a physiological-function standpoint. Discussion with the psychotherapist may be very important; at times therapy needs to be put on hold until the depression is brought under control.

Borderline personality disorder

What a horrible name for a condition that is! It makes the patient think of herself as not quite a person. And BPD patients are treated that way, too: as pariahs, socially, in family life, at work, and in the doctor's office.

There is a large overlap: about 60 percent of patients who are dissociative also fit the criteria for BPD. (On the other hand, it does not go the other way, with 60 percent of borderline personality patients being dissociative.) The reason for the overlap is not hard to find: both stem from the same source—growing up in a highly dysfunctional family. I usually explain to them, to ease their mortification when they are told about the coexisting diagnosis (as one does for assessment purposes, for example) that they simply did not have the opportunity to learn good coping skills when they were small so they are still coping the way they did when they were five years old. Thus, part of the task of therapy is for them to learn new, better ways of coping.

It's an uphill struggle. BPD patients are inevitably cast as manipulative, domineering, demanding, exasperating, and not wanting to get well. All of those apply, except the last one: in fact, they are fiercely anxious to get well. Unfortunately, they haven't learned or understood that getting well is their job and not ours. Ours is to help them; we can't do it for them. As we pursue the goal with them, it is our job to manage our own countertransference. And that may be a challenge!

Suicide and self-harm

As there is usually one ego state who is very depressed, there is also usually one ego state who frequently appears to be suicidal. It may not be the depressed part, but instead a part who truly believes that it would be best for "Mary" (the host) if she were dead and Mary is somehow convinced of the appropriateness of this decision.

Let us look first at the depressed part. Calls from the emergency room to say that the patient has been brought in as a probable suicide attempt are certainly not rare. Such attempts are seldom fatal, however. I think the other parts of the system prevent the suicidal one from carrying out the plan. It is even more common for an ego state who assumes the role of informer to phone and tell you that Mary is planning to kill herself that evening. This call comes, of course, just as you are getting ready to go out to dinner. (All this is avoided for the family physician if the patient calls the therapist, instead, in these situations. You can encourage this. It is not being nasty: it is being realistic. Probably the therapist has better skills than the family physician in dealing with suicidal ideation.)

Staying in the hospital overnight is probably a good idea. The patient is safe, it gives a breathing period, and the other parts of the personality can come to the fore. It must be addressed, however. Otherwise, it is still simmering under the surface and the protectors in the system will come to the conclusion that you don't care.

There is another aspect that appears to be suicidal but in reality is a plan to kill a suffering ego state, in the belief that it will do her a favor, as we saw a little earlier. You may be astonished at how difficult it is to persuade the ego state who is advocating this action, that she (the advocate) would die also. "I'm not her" is the response. It only confirms how disparate their sense of self really is.

Self-harm is also a common feature of dissociative disorders, although it is not so prominent in PTSD. Cutting is the main form, but hitting and burning with cigarettes are also frequently found. The rationale is always the same: "It lets the pain out." The patients always heal well and quickly, often with no medical intervention at all. There is a book called *A Bright Red Scream* (Strong, 1998), which is about self-harm through cutting. I think the title explains it very well.

Patients are often very embarrassed to confess to the self-harm, believing that we will despise them. Here is one place where the family physician can be truly helpful to the patient. Listen carefully, take her seriously, and have a conversation about it. Be sure that the patient knows you do not think less of her, that you do realize how difficult it was to tell you about it and that it helps you to understand how deep her emotional pain really is.

Dangerous sexual practices exemplify a different type of self-harm. This may involve prostitution, unprotected sex, or gang involvement, among other behaviors. STDs, assaults, extreme abuse (including deliberate harm to the genitalia and/or unwanted pregnancies, and perhaps attempts to self-abort) ensue. If possible, talk to the patient's therapist about these kinds of activity and work together if you can. It is usually one ego state who indulges in sexual danger.

Alcohol abuse

Of all the substance abuse found with dissociative patients, alcoholism is probably the one most frequently encountered.

It presents in a variety of ways. It is not uncommon for the system to have one ego state that is alcoholic and the rest of the ego states not. This can create havoc in both patient and her family, as you can imagine—everything from denial of using alcohol at all, which the rest of the ego states are eager to make clear, to law-breaking activity while under the influence of liquor.

The "alcoholic" ego state may be a teenager bent on trying out the world, or a depressed part looking for solace, or a rebel determined to break as many moral restrictions as possible.

On the other hand, alcoholism in someone with PTSD or DDNOS may have an entirely different basis, such as the need to block out disturbing images and memories. It doesn't work, of course, but it is a very common route to take in a search for peace.

Apparently, there is a much greater risk factor with those who have histories of severe abuse in early childhood. Such survivors (if you choose to use that term) have a four- to twelve-times greater risk of developing alcoholism, depression, drug abuse, and suicide attempts than the general population according to some researchers, and a two- to four-times greater risk of smoking (Felitti et al, 1998).

The explanation is that interpersonal trauma, especially when one is very young and with those who are supposed to care for one, makes one vulnerable to developing "emotion-focused coping"— a coping style geared to a persistent concern about one's immediate emotional state—rather than focusing on the circumstances that produce those states. (There is now a new therapeutic approach utilizing this concept.) This type of focus is associated with a high rate (25–40 percent) of alcohol and substance abuse (McFarlane, 2001).

As one might surmise, the relationship between substance abuse and PTSD is reciprocal: drug abuse leads to exposure to traumatic events while exposure to trauma leads to substance use. It is estimated that between a quarter and a half of all patients who seek substance-abuse treatment suffer from a comorbid PTSD and/or dissociative disorder (van der Kolk, 2003).

To reiterate:

- comorbidity is very common with dissociative disorders
- we need to carefully differentiate between depression in a single ego state and depression as a central diagnosis
- suicide ideation and self-harm are common and also have to be differentiated as to the source
- substance abuse is also common, especially with alcohol, and can seriously interfere with the patient's psychotherapy.

Chapter Ten
Body-Image Distortions

According to van der Kolk et al. (1996), it is affect dysregulation—an inability to understand one's emotions and emotional responses—that is the source of the sometimes stunning distortions of self-image that one finds with dissociative patients.

By now it will not be any news to you that the various ego states present in distinctly different ways—different mode of dress, different ways of speaking, of posture, of general presentation, which become easily recognizable after we get to know the patient a little better and it feels safe for him to allow us to recognize the separateness that he believes exists between the different parts of his personality structure.

We know that there are all ages of ego states, as well as males and females and sometimes nonhumans (robots or animals), and that each part has a different role to play in its interactions with the outside world. Sometimes they are of different race.

These various parts of the self are seen, from inside, to be distinct and appear as different as two people in the outside world would appear. In a complex DID patient, of course, they don't all know each other, and as the amnesia barriers are gradually and gently erased ("dismantled" is the term used), she may come into the office one day, somewhat mystified, and describe the stranger that she saw last night, cooking the dinner in her very own kitchen. When she looks in the mirror, the various parts are seen to appear distinctly different, and that includes when she looks into her "inside mirror". If you ask her to draw some of her ego states, the drawings will appear to be a group of strangers rather than the person you know and see.

Van der Kolk et al. (1996) describe this affect regulation as a "lack of self-regulatory processes [which are] likely to have a profound effect … on the sense of self, such as a sense of separateness and disturbances of body image". I interpret this to mean that, because the person has never learned how to keep his emotional response contained and directed appropriately, it is instead directed in "parts", which mirror the emotion itself. I alluded to the nature of ego states as being linked to emotional response in the Introduction (page xi). Furthermore, the patient feels that he has absolutely no control over the other ego states in the system.

I must qualify that last statement. Very often, as psychotherapy proceeds, a kind of hierarchy is revealed, congruent with the role that the ego state plays in the system. This makes sense, when one considers the child parts, for example. One of Jayere's child parts seemed to her to be definitely connected to her in some way that the other parts were not, so we called that part "Jayce", meaning J.C.—"Jayere's Child". She was a very sweet ego state, which I think was reflective of the child that Jayere had hoped to be, but because of the extremely strict discipline in the house, felt that she had never achieved.

The depersonalization that many dissociative patients experience is another example of these distortions of body image. In a depersonalization situation, they experience themselves to be not real. They may also have the sense that their hands or feet are getting larger or in some other way changing in size or shape. To feel "not real"—one's sense of self cannot get more distorted than that.

Eating disorders, especially anorexia, exemplify body-image distortions to the nth degree. When she looks in the mirror, all she sees is a fat, ugly female—not even worthy of being called a girl or woman, just a female.

At times there is a belief that one or more ego states come from a past life. The role of such a part is usually to advise and protect, perhaps as an old crone, or a warrior, but I have met a destructive saboteur, too, determined to rid this world of a scourge from the past. Understanding that every ego state first comes to fulfill a need, I struggle with the implications of such a part of the self. Might this be a source of some deep depression? Perhaps, but I think the psychological ramifications of such a self-belief might be manifested in physical symptoms. If you have a patient with, say, many aspects of DDNOS, and also of somatoform expression, you may find it interesting to inquire, in a very supportive way, as to the patient's sense of what purpose or role his symptoms serve, making it clear that you want to understand better so that the two of you can collaborate in finding more useful remedies, be they psychological or medical or a little of both.

To reiterate:

- distortions in body image are almost universal in dissociative patients
- having patients draw or describe their ego states, clarifies the ways in which they perceive themselves
- eating-disorder patients have a bizarre belief that they are fat and ugly
- amnesia barriers often exist between the ego states.

Chapter Eleven
Eating Disorders

Eating disorders, especially anorexia and bulimia, are classic examples of what I call "contained" dissociative disorders. The dissociation is expressed primarily in one part of the patient's life (although sequelae, such as sexual dysfunction, often brim over into other areas). Seldom are the ego states strangers to one another. At the same time, the patient is (or believes herself to be) powerless to challenge or deny the part (or parts) of herself that demands this incredibly bizarre behavior.

Eating disorders occur in boys and men too, but by far the majority of them are seen in women. (This gave rise to the oft-repeated assumption that anorexia occurs because the girl is too highly influenced by the fashion magazines and peer pressure. It is not nearly as simple as that.) For the sake of expediency, I'll refer to the patients, in this chapter, as "she" (I have, anyway, been "sharing out" the personal pronouns between the genders), recognizing that I am therefore apparently ignoring those suffering males who also have severe eating disorders. Please believe me: I am not ignoring them. I know that they are in agony also.

Elisha was referred to me by her pediatrician, in the hope that some hypnosis might help her deal with her problems more effectively. She was seventeen when I met her—a sweet, gentle girl who sat as far into the corner in my office as she was able to reach.

Her family history, which she told me haltingly over several appointments, was of a very physically abusive mother and an older sexually abusive brother. She was sure that, when she told me about the brother, I would be so disgusted with her as a person that I would tell her to leave my office, that I couldn't treat such an evil girl. I have a hard time imagining the courage it must have taken for her to disclose this history to me, all the while believing that I would utterly reject her. (In adult years, the brother admitted to these abuses.) She did not have the same concerns when telling me about the mother, believing that she deserved the extremely harsh punishment which was meted out to her on a daily basis.

As she arrived into her teens, the punishment stopped, and she and her mother eventually worked through the memories of these terrible parts of their lives. Elisha was infinitely forgiving, saying, "It calmed her to beat me. It made her feel better." Nevertheless, she finally did come to the realization that she was *not* a very, very bad girl but that her mother had severe psychological problems of her own.

At seventeen, Elisha was able to attend to the sexual abuse and we spent our first few months in the therapy sessions, working on this. The therapy proceeded fairly smoothly, once I was able to convince her that I found her admirable rather than disgusting. That took some time, and it was with great wariness that she first began to accept it.

Her own family physician, a woman whom she liked and who liked her, nevertheless asked me to take Elisha into my own family practice, as my colleague felt overwhelmed by the problems Elisha presented to her. I did so, after ascertaining that Elisha wanted this also. In fact, it cemented her growing belief that I did find her an acceptable human being, for which she was thankful. She seldom, though, came for problems unrelated to the anorexia and/or specific work on abuse issues.

Elisha was the one who taught me about the essential dissociative nature of anorexia and bulimia. She told me about the voices, she told me about the absolute sense that she had no control over the voices and what they told her to do, even though she knew full well what was happening. She told me about the incredible abdominal pain, produced by horrendous doses of laxatives, and how she had to be careful to go to different drug stores so that no one would suspect.

I reassured her, over and over, that she was not crazy.

It took years, but she recovered. This is far more a testament to her than to my therapeutic skills, because she was the teacher, I the pupil. She is now happily married, to a sensitive man who allowed her to take her time with intimacy. Although I am no longer in family practice, we keep in touch with Christmas cards and the occasional postcard.

Where is the source of the problem?

Not all anorexia/bulimia patients have a history of sexual abuse. I want to make that very clear. However, attachment theory certainly plays a role here. Neither does that mean that the parents do not love their child. In many cases, they do and always have done. Nevertheless, something has gone off track, somewhere. And it is important to recognize that abuse is in the background of many of these patients. One patient knew all the tricks to pretend to eat, but managed to stay as thin as a rail. I was always bemused that her mother was thin as a rail, too, although she was certainly very worried about her daughter. (I did not mean that in a sarcastic way.)

Generally, they have always been very *good* children, always thinking of others first and doing whatever they can to be helpful around the house. "Altogether *too* perfect," one of my colleagues once growled to me, when discussing a case. Indeed, in families where, for example, the mother might be having problems, the child will often become the caregiver. They are good students, too, and their teachers love them.

Often the young girl will be slightly chubby (again giving rise to the "influenced by fashion" theory). She will start dieting, go to the gym, become nice and trim. Everyone will compliment her. But then she becomes extremely slim, then thin, and often, eventually, skeletal. Strangely, her health usually remains generally good. Other patients, though, have no history of chubbiness, so that that cannot be used as one of the predisposing factors, or certainly not in every case.

Then the tendency is to begin equating thinness with goodness. And the inner voices begin to take control. Soon, they rule her life. She is helpless against them; she must do what they tell her to do.

The voices tell her that she is no good; that she doesn't deserve to eat, or even deserve to be alive; that she is worthless as a human being. Perhaps, if she gets a little thinner, she may redeem herself to her voices—except that it doesn't work that way and they keep on berating her. They tell her that she is not allowed to eat or that, if she does, she must exercise into exhaustion and/or consume huge qualities of laxatives to get rid of the food as quickly as possible. Many patients make themselves vomit after eating, even small amounts. (In general, anorexia is when the patient refuses to eat anything; bulimia is when she eats and then purges or vomits. Of course, this is also too simplistic and many cases are combinations of these two aspects.)

Bulimia versus anorexia

Bulimic patients often maintain a reasonable weight, as opposed to anorexic patients, because they do eat and at least some nutritional elements get absorbed. Also, the bulimic may (and often does) binge first and then purge, so she may take in significantly more calories than the anorexia patient. And one does not always find the "very good little girl" history that is so frequently present in the anorexic patient.

Because of the bingeing, the bulimic patient may have a different (but still very important) type of self-disgust: she may hate herself for the bingeing, be very self-condemnatory because of what she perceives to be the lack of willpower.

In contrast, the true anorexic will eat almost nothing. She might, however, cook for others, enjoy making fancy meals or desserts and encouraging the family to eat them. It seems to me to be a terrible kind of vicarious gustatory pleasure.

This is dissociation—in spades. Treatment and recovery without attending to the dissociative aspect is, I believe, virtually hopeless. The voices are her ego states. They are not logical. They reflect some very deep inner turmoil of which she has no understanding, let alone an explanation as to its purpose.

She gets thinner. Her parents are becoming very worried, but she isn't—not at all. Indeed, it is taken as a sign that she is achieving her goal: she is becoming thinner and, *ipso facto*, better. She is the quintessential *"la belle indifference"* about the weight loss, and she still believes herself to be fat.

Because she is a very good girl, always concerned about the feelings of others, she will often pretend to eat; then she may cache food, in her lap or a napkin, or under the table for the family pet. Or hold it in her mouth, excuse herself to go to the bathroom, and spit it out.

When she goes to the doctor, she will often tie weights around her waist or in her clothes so that the extreme weight loss does not show on the scale. Of course, she will refuse to get undressed and the doctor is loath to force her, especially in these litigious days. Heavy shoes are another ploy.

Potential complications

Despite the overt appearance of calm, she may be extremely suicidal, and this is something that the family doctor needs to address specifically. Delaying a straight discussion may end up being too late. Antidepressants, in my experience, are often of little help.

She may also self-injure, and this is a fairly frequent complication. Again, it drives the parents to distraction and the girl is worried not at all. "It just helps," she might say. "It seems to let some of the pain out." Or, her voices tell her to do it, and she does.

Endocrinologically, because she is so thin her menses usually stop and her libido is greatly depressed. Once more harking back to old rationales, this was taken as a sign that she really just wanted to stay a little girl for ever. I believe that this, also, is too simplistic. It has to do with an extremely distorted body image, not a wish to remain a little girl.

Bulimic patients may have evidence of vomiting or purging: discolored teeth, a quite specific halitosis, esophagitis, reflux. A barium swallow may possibly be in order if she is complaining of epigastric pain. The anus may be extremely irritated because of the laxative-induced diarrhea.

What can you do?

Explain that you need to do a full physical examination to make sure that there are not some physical reasons for her extreme thinness. She may want her mother in the room when you do this, or she may absolutely *not* want her mother in the room. In all events, make sure that the nurse is present (mother or no mother). Record your clinical findings meticulously, and your observations regarding mood and compliance, also.

Share your findings with her—alone, if she is of age.

Tell her that you know about the voices, and that you also know that she is not crazy. Explain that there is a part (or are parts) of her that wants to influence her about eating and becoming thin, and that you know she finds it (or them) very powerful. And reassure her that *she* is powerful, too, and that she can learn to be just as powerful as the voices are. She won't believe you, but tell her anyway, and many times.

Tell her that you, as her family doctor, are always going to be interested in her wellbeing and will do your best to keep her well.

Keep notes about your observations, so that you can pass them along to appropriate people.

What can you **not** do?

You can't treat this yourself, unless you are trained and experienced in the treatment of dissociative disorders. Even then, it's difficult. Explain that you are going to help her find a therapist who will, in turn, help her to understand more about the voices, and that the therapist will not think that she is crazy, either. Your local psychological association may be able to suggest an appropriate therapist, or you may wish to contact the International Society for the Study of Dissociation or one of its component societies in the U.K., Canada, or other countries.

Some areas have eating-disorder clinics within the hospital setting. These are almost universally detested by the patients, who view them as coercive and otherwise unhelpful.

These units may employ force-feeding or extreme consequences, such as not allowing any visitors, unless the patient eats what is presented to her. Almost invariably the patient will find a way to get rid of the food.

In the long run, most anorexic patients put on enough weight in the hospital so that they will be discharged, and then go right back to their own determination to be thin. This is not so hard to understand: in the hospital, nothing has really changed. Of course, there are units where good psychotherapy is part of the plan, and these are in a different category.

There are some private clinics around, most of which charge very high fees. They have a different perspective about the treatment of eating disorders, especially anorexia and bulimia (and we have to remember that extreme obesity is an eating disorder, too). Some of these clinics have the patient as an inpatient for a very long time, and have someone with her constantly to make sure that she does not exercise in secret, for instance, or throw up.

Part of the reason these private clinics are so expensive is that they require a huge staff to maintain the constant surveillance, staying with the patient even during the sleeping hours. Some of them are internationally known and attract desperate families from all over the world.

There is a fairly extensive literature about eating disorders, often found in the literature of the dissociative disorders. See Chapter Seventeen for some examples.

To reiterate: when you have an eating-disorder patient, look for:

- family factors, which *may* include a history of abuse
- attempts to hide weights in clothing
- self-harm
- suicidal ideation
- the "very good girl" personality
- cessation of menses and/or decreased libido
- evidence of purging or vomiting
- apparent compliance if hospitalized, then a quick reversion to the anorexic state
- an extremely negative self-image (despite the "good girl" façade).

Chapter Twelve
Sleep Disturbances

Looking at those charts on pages 43 and 44 again (which by now you may never want to see again), you will see that sleep disturbances are common in all the chronic syndromes as well as PTSD and the other dissociative disorders. Indeed, it is often the kind of thing that brings the patient into the family physician's office.

As always, we need to take a thorough history. When, where, how, and why did the poor sleeping patterns get established? What else was going on in your life at the time? (This question is seldom answered accurately in this context.) Do you have trouble *getting* to sleep, or *staying* asleep? If you waken during the night, how long does it take you to get back to sleep?

While you are asking the questions, look for shifts in body language, eye contact and speech tone and language. Often, if there is a dissociative disorder, there will be some switching of ego states and this may give you some clue as to the root of the problem.

Flashbacks and nightmares

People with PTSD often have flashbacks in their sleep. They may not even waken the patient, who finds himself drenched with sweat when he does rouse. At that time, there is often a feeling of doom, but the person has no clue why, or what has happened. The flashback is often not remembered.

Of course, it may also be that the flashback does waken the person, who suddenly comes alert and finds himself terrified and back in the jungle, or under the train, or being attacked by the mugger/rapist/wild animal. These dreadful experiences are also terrifying for the spouse or partner, who wakens too, and who seems unable to do anything to soothe or calm the patient, or even bring the person back into the present. It is an awful feeling, not to be able to help someone you love who is obviously in horrible distress.

So how can you help? You can help by teaching both patient and spouse the basic grounding techniques: *"Breathe!* You are here, at home [give address—street, town, (and country if the patient is a war vet)]. Look at me. I am here with you [give your name] and I will stay with you. [repeat this several times]. *Breathe!* Look around you. See [the clock, the TV, the cat—whatever you can find to normalize and familiarize the place]. Feel the rug [floor, tile] under your feet. Feel its warmth [coolness]. *Breathe!"*

Sometimes a cool cloth on the forehead or back of the neck, or a sip of cold water, will help to bring the person back. On the other hand, if he has been sweating profusely, a warm blanket over the shoulders may be more appropriate to prevent the chills.

Sleep flashbacks may be silent, or noisy with shouts and cries and wails and foul language. It may be important to explain to youngsters in the house, so that they are not also thrust into fear.

As I explained in a previous chapter, nightmares are to flashbacks what memory is to dissociation: in the one, there is a distinct separation from the present time and place, i.e. the person is back in the trauma situation; in the other, it is recognized as a nightmare or memory, albeit a nasty one, and the person is oriented in time and place when he wakes.

Anxiety and/or depression

Anxiety is often the cause of sleep problems (not only for those who have a dissociative disorder, of course). This may vary from "What if I can never get to sleep all night?" (a sure way to keep oneself awake) to "What if something happens to me in the night and I never wake up? What if there's a fire? What if …" (you name it).

However, having a terrified ego state is a little bit different, and is really quite common in someone who has a dissociative disorder—not necessarily DID, because DDNOS patients seem to be equally affected. It is surely not hard to understand that such an entity might be present—in fact, it is rare for one not to be present somewhere in the system.

If this seems to be the case, it may be useful to talk to the patient's therapist (as always, with permission). He or she may be able to organize a Helper ego state to take care of the terrified one at nighttime/bedtime. If you have a good rapport with the patient, you may even approach this yourself, but usually it is best coming from the therapist. If you do decide to approach it yourself, some simple phrase such as "Could we ask a helping part of you who can, and would be willing to, comfort the young one who seems to be so frightened, so that every one can get comfortably to sleep?"

On the other hand, it might just be straight anxiety, not necessarily a young child part. The question then becomes, what is the best way to deal with the anxiety? Many patients will ask for pills; you'll have to make up your own mind as to whether it is appropriate to prescribe. If you do, I would suggest (again) one of the tricyclics in a small dose, rather than an anxiolytic. If sleep is seriously impaired, such that the person cannot carry on with his usual daily activities or go to work, that gets put onto the balance scales. Many physicians are more comfortable with SSRIs than with the older tricyclics—if this is you, again look at a small dose.

This changes somewhat if you are looking at anxiety masking as depression. Decisions again. Is the depression interfering with normal sleep patterns? Is the patient sleeping too much, rather than too little? In such a case, something like paroxetine may indeed be indicated. Sometimes we forget that patients with dissociative disorders are people, after all, like everybody else, and deserve to be considered for themselves rather than their DSM-IV diagnosis.

Perhaps this patient has a chronic pain syndrome? Sleep disturbances are common. You will remember that it is a vicious cycle:

pain leads to poor sleep, which leads to the formation of Substance P, which leads to more pain, which leads to … and on and on. This cycle really does need to be interrupted. Personally, I teach hypnotic pain relief and sleep-beckoning techniques. If you yourself do not do hypnosis, enlist the help of a colleague. It almost always works if the patient is comfortable with the idea of hypnosis and doesn't fear that some one is taking over his mind.

Nighttime activity

It is not at all uncommon for dissociative patients to complain that they are always tired when they get up in the morning, and then they find that somehow, during the night, the ironing got done and the living room was vacuumed. Or that letter to Aunt Nellie somehow got written (it had been postponed so many times, yet there it was).

The answer is obvious—some other part of the system was up, doing the chores. (At other times, the chores get done and yet nobody is tired—an equally mystifying phenomenon!) In such cases, it may cause more distress to the spouse than to the patient.

It is part of the bewildering physiology of the dissociative patient. Of course, it happens when there are strong amnesia barriers between ego states, and one part literally does not know what another part is doing or has done.

What can you do?

Well, perhaps nothing, unless the patient is distressed. Is the tiredness sufficient to be worrying or may a little reassurance that he is healthy be all that is needed? Here is another occasion where you can talk in a straightforward manner to the patient if there is good rapport regarding the dissociation. If there is no particular problem to the patient, except perhaps a little irritation that things are going on that he does not remember doing (although is glad to have them done), then there is no harm and nothing to really worry about. Just be amazed, as I so often am, at the incredible resilience and creativity that is part and parcel of dissociation.

To reiterate:

- sleep disturbances are common in trauma-spectrum disorders
- careful differentiation between what is troublesome and what is not usually answers the question of whether intervention is necessary
- flashbacks, nightmares, anxiety and/or depression, terror or another ego state's activity almost always accounts for the sleep disturbance
- chronic pain syndromes have one more item in the differential diagnosis—release of more Substance P.

Chapter Thirteen
Sexual Dysfunction

I had met Mrs. A. before, when she had come for some pain-management techniques for her chronic pelvic-pain syndrome. (She was adamantly opposed to the designation "Ms.", so I'll continue with "Mrs." out of respect for her feelings.)

This time, she came with her husband, and the presenting complaint was dyspareunia. That didn't seem very different from chronic pelvic-pain syndrome, so I asked about that.

Mr. A. interrupted as she had started to answer. "No, this is different," he insisted, "because it interrupts our sex life. In fact, it pretty well eliminates our sex life. And she never has a climax—it's as if nothing can make that happen."

I turned to her and asked, "How is the pain different?" Then, as he again began to interrupt, I said, "No, please let her answer herself, in her own words."

She spoke haltingly. "I don't know, really, except that it just hurts so much when he—he—"

"Enters?" I suggested.

"Yes. And then when he … pushes, you know?"

"Yes, I understand. And this is different, apparently, from the pain that you have had for so long in your pelvis. Because this pain only happens with intercourse?"

"Yes." A whisper.

"And the other pain? Is it still there?"

"Oh, yes, it's always there, but it seems to be like a constant ache, whereas this—this is more of a—a—a stabbing pain." She gasped at the implication.

Her husband shifted in his chair. "Honey, you know that I never want to hurt you, but—"

"Oh, yes, I know that, of course. But I don't know what to do. I just can't stand this other pain, when we're ... together." She was weeping.

In a matter-of-fact way, I explained that I would need to examine her, and my nurse would show her to the examination room. Then I said to them both that we would need to talk some more. Her husband told her that he would just go off and do some errands, and would return for her in half an hour. Some of the lines of worry on her face smoothed out, so I didn't interfere with alternative suggestions.

Again, in a matter-of-fact way, I weighed her, took her blood pressure, listened to heart and lungs. Palpation of the abdomen was normal—no visceromegaly or masses, soft, generally non-tender, good bowel sounds. She had relaxed a bit, but tensed up again and I explained that I would do a routine pelvic exam including a PAP smear.

"What did the gynecologists tell you?" I asked. I knew that she had had at least two referrals for the chronic pelvic-pain problem.

She bit her lip. "Both of them told me that I was impossible to examine," she said. "They made it sound as if it was all my fault."

"Well, we're not having too much of a problem today, are we? Just breathe some relaxation right *here*, if you please." I pressed with my gloved fingers at the introitus. Rather unexpectedly, she did. "Good!" I encouraged her.

The initial stages of the pelvic exam proceeded fairly smoothly. I took the PAP and reported to her that the cervix and vagina looked healthy. Then, removing the speculum, I began the bimanual exam, when to my complete astonishment, she had a major orgasm.

"I won't examine you any more today," I told her gently. She was crying as if her heart would break. And later, back in my consulting room, she continued to cry—torrents of tears. After several minutes, it abated.

"Please, don't tell my husband," she begged. "Please, please don't tell him."

"Help me to understand what's going on here," I responded.

The story came out haltingly, in phrases and half-sentences, more tears, then a few more words. When we—together—deciphered it all, it turned out that she had been sexually abused as a teenager; her parents had berated her cruelly and told her that she was worthless and a disgrace to the family (although she had been held down so that she couldn't escape), and the message was loud and clear that she was a tramp. Apparently, the worst abuse came when she was accused of enjoying the sex. "And the awful, the really *awful*, part was that I think maybe I *did*." She stopped, again overcome with emotion.

With adolescent agony, and unable to find any counterargument to the statement that no nice girl ever *enjoyed* it, she swore that she would never again allow herself to reach sexual satisfaction.

Consequently, during sexual encounters she was rigid with tension, the vaginismus alone enough to prevent all but the most determined partner, and if penetration was, somehow, achieved, the emotional agony was translated by her body into extreme dyspareunia.

The subsequent therapeutic journey was long and very difficult for her. She had never told her husband of the old experience, believing that, if she did, he would completely reject her. Some part of herself told her that this somehow didn't make sense, but the emotional ego states took over and kept flipping her back to her adolescent self.

Of course, Mrs. A. was not a major dissociative disorder. Nevertheless, her childhood had been difficult in that home life was always rife with strident conflict. Her mother told all the children, but particularly Mrs. A and her sister, that women were just men's pawns, that childbirth was ghastly and no baby was worth it. The disattachment is blatant. When she was sexually attacked, she "went away" in her imagination (a dissociative coping mechanism), and she told me that she had often used that capability when the family raged around her.

I wondered aloud whether she did this when she and her husband were being intimate. She told me that she had tried to do that, but somehow she always found herself back at the time of the sexual assault, which didn't seem very helpful.

Abuse, dissociation and sexual dysfunction

All types of abuse—emotional, physical, and sexual—can lead to sexual dysfunction. That dysfunction can, in turn, assume many guises and presentations.

Anorgasmia is common. Dyspareunia, vaginismus and pelvic-pain syndrome are the other problems most often encountered. But the true dissociative patient presents unique variations on the common themes.

Consider this. A couple come to the family doctor's office for joint counseling around sexual problems. When asked to describe those problems, it becomes quickly apparent that the husband is very distressed and completely confused. He believes that it must be his fault, because his wife is otherwise loving—most of the time—and tender toward him. But, as soon as he approaches her sexually, she withdraws, sometimes coldly and with anger.

At first, he thought it must be all his fault. Then he began to believe that it is all *her* fault. He feels confused, angry and rejected.

When asked, the wife responds that, most of the time, she just doesn't feel like it. She's tired, she has lots to do the next day, she needs her sleep.

Or consider this. The husband, confused and angry, says that sometimes his wife is so sexually welcoming that he almost feels attacked, yet at other times she practically turns on him if he even mentions it, and—worst of all—there are times when she invites the lovemaking, then in the middle she turns on him, even hits him, or—my God!—acts as if she were three years old!

Women (and men) with dissociative disorders may have ego states that are seductive, or promiscuous, or childlike, or cold. Typically, the "good wife" ego state is appalled at the thought that, at times, she leaves the house and picks up some stranger on the street. She may not even know that she does this, but is told that she was seen or she finds other evidence of it in the form of a hotel receipt or unaccountable money in her purse.

Both male and female patients may have homosexual or bisexual ego states, which may further confuse the issue.

Physiologically, the women are usually healthy, with normal hormonal function and parameters. Anatomically they are normal, too.

However, there may be unexplained sexually transmitted diseases with a very strange response to the usual medications. Bizarre as it seems, one ego state may have the infection and another not. And, if you tell me that that is impossible, I will agree with you—and tell you that there is documented evidence of this when vaginal swabs were taken twenty minutes apart. One came back with no pathological infection, the other was positive for chlamydia (one of my own patients told me disdainfully, "Of course, I don't have it, *she* does"). Other family physicians with dissociative patients have had the same experiences.

I wish somebody could explain this to me, because I can't explain it to myself. However, it may provide the answer for some beleaguered family doc who can't understand why the treatment isn't working, or seemed to work just fine and then the problem came back again, apparently overnight.

Men who are dissociative have frequently been viciously attacked anally, or the penis has been deliberately and painfully harmed. Erectile dysfunction is a frequent consequence. Men also may have seductive, loving, promiscuous or violent ego states. Drug abuse is common, too. Also, many dissociative males have formed the conclusion in childhood that sexual encounters are always violent, rapelike, with no interest or consideration for the partner (male or female).

There is an understandable tendency to attribute all sexual dysfunction to child abuse. Obviously, this is just as bad as refusing to consider that child abuse has any bearing on the problem at all. But some patients just need good therapy to help them find their own *adult* sexuality. It may be that there have been events in childhood that were confusing—although not abusive—such as hearing the parents making strange noises during the night. Or something happened in school—it could have been a teacher's comment, or other children pontificating about something they really knew nothing about and were very inaccurate in describing; or that old standby, television, bringing strange and disturbing images into a young person's mind. Or there may have been, or still were, anatomical and/or physiological reasons why sexual activity was frightening or painful. We always need to keep things in perspective, and inquire patiently, skillfully and open-mindedly about the roots of sexual dysfunction.

What can you do?

Be aware of the possibility of dissociativity when sexual problems arise and appear to be somehow incongruent with the circumstances.

It is all right to ask openly about what the patient's growing-up years were like. Ask also about any history of sexual abuse, at any age. (Helpful hint: if the patient says, "Oh, my childhood was wonderful!" and then cannot remember any of it, you may perhaps be a bit wary of believing that it was all *that* wonderful.)

Attend to the physical health concerns—STDs, AIDS, etc.— diligently. Be sure to do annual PAP smears. Take note of inconsistent histories, or of one partner saying everything is fine and the other near to despair.

All sexual orientations are vulnerable to sexual dysfunctions.

Depending on the circumstances, it may or may not be appropriate to refer the patient. Perhaps the problem is best handled by the family doctor, in whom the patient has a degree of trust. If it comes to psychotherapy, of course, referral is the appropriate course. If it has to do with managing the problem of the day, and that has to do with health issues, then most family physicians are in a good position to take care of it. Just keep a clear view and an open mind.

To reiterate: when you have a patient with inexplicable or recurring sexual problems, ask yourself:

- could this be explained by some degree of dissociativity?
- would this answer some of the confusing aspects?
- check for STDs
- check for AIDS
- do annual PAPs, even on teenagers and older women
- remember that chronic pelvic-pain syndrome may be associated with dissociativity.

Chapter Fourteen
Relationships

Karl and Carla had been married for twelve years—and stormy years they had been. They had lost many friends because of the battles that had been waged in public, and their three daughters had been embarrassed more than once because of their parents' disruptive behavior.

Although both, along with their children, were patients in my family practice, I seldom saw Karl. I had delivered all of the children, and seen them through the early years of colic, teething, toddling, and vaccinations, heard about their first days at kindergarten and into elementary school and knew them to be intelligent and outgoing. I wondered at their mother's somewhat cavalier attitude at times, but she certainly seemed to be a very caring mother. She seldom spoke about her husband.

The eldest girl, about the time she turned ten, seemed to be becoming more withdrawn. However, she was doing well at school, according to all reports, and her mother didn't offer any comments regarding the apparent shift from happy-go-lucky to silent and downcast.

I was surprised, therefore, to begin noticing something else about Carla. As the children grew a little older (they were now six, eight, and ten) she herself seemed to be growing somewhat distant from them, even from the youngest. One day when the youngest child and her mother were in to see about eye testing for the little girl, I asked Carla if anything else was bothering her about the children.

"Not about the children," she snapped, in a voice I hadn't heard before. "It's about their idiot of a father."

Hearing that, the little girl began to cry.

"Let's go look and see if there's a new puzzle," I said to the child and, finding one, added, "Now you see how well you can fit those pieces together and Mommy and I will just talk for a few minutes." She nodded, snuffling her tears.

When I turned to look at Carla again, she was smiling brightly, not with the waspish face I had seen a few moments before. "Things going all right at home?" I asked.

"Sure, just fine," she replied. "Why?"

"I thought you sounded a bit stressed a few minutes ago," I said.

She looked confused for a brief moment. "Why?" she asked again.

"And Cheryl looked a bit distressed, too," I continued.

She started to cry. "I don't know what's wrong," she said. "Karl accuses me of things that I never said or did, and he seems determined to make me believe that I did them—things I would never think of doing. I just don't understand it." She wiped the tears away. "Anyhow, who cares?" she threw out defiantly. "He's just a jerk."

She wasn't very enthusiastic when I suggested that she and Karl might come into the office sometime and talk about their ups and downs, but said she'd think about it. After she had left, however, *I* started to think about it.

By that time I had already recognized another dissociative patient in the practice (Jayere) and had begun to work with two or three others who had been referred to me. I looked back on the previous few years through a different lens, and thought I recognized a pattern.

Sure enough, I had.

Karl was defensive and Carla was bitter when they came in together. As the story unfolded—the inconsistent behavior, the apparent lies, and the erratic moods—he looked miserable. Carla didn't offer any explanations, just glared from time to time; however, once or twice, I saw a glisten of tears. I began, slowly and carefully, to share my thoughts. "I've been wondering—" I said, and as I continued to speak I saw a sudden and unmistakable shift in Carla.

"You better know what you're talking about," she said, almost snarling.

I nodded. "Yes," I rejoined, "I think I do."

Over the next few weeks we worked our way through the various diagnostic tools, and I heard more history from both sides, including details of Carla's young years that I had never heard before. As the true picture emerged, Karl looked so relieved that my heart went out to him. "I was truly thinking of leaving," he said. "Now that I understand what's been happening, of course I'll stay. We'll see it through together."

The said fact is that relationships are incredibly difficult to maintain when one partner is dissociative. Not only are there the apparent wild mood swings, but there are almost always sexual difficulties, such as have been described earlier, that make spousal life even more difficult. Of course we must remember that at times it is the husband whose personality is in compartments and the wife who is at her wits' end. For various reasons, though, this situation may be less intrusive, as his behavior can always be explained by having to work late at the office; he usually isn't the main child care-giver; he goes to watch the ball game and she doesn't like sports anyhow; and similar plausible excuses.

It isn't hard to figure out why these problems emerge. Marriage, or sharing life with a partner, depends on being able to *trust*. And trusting is the hardest thing in the world to do, for someone who has had the kind of childhood experiences that virtually all significantly dissociative people have had. How can you trust, when you have learned from a very early age that trusting is dangerous? How can you trust when you have learned also that trusting people whom you are supposed to be *able* to trust is especially dangerous because those are the people who hurt you or who have not protected you from danger and/or being hurt?

It all has to do with poor attachments—that is, not being able to rely on another person to be there for you when you need it. If that crucial capacity to be able rely on and trust a close family member or friend has not been instilled when we are very young, it is excruciatingly difficult to learn it when we are adults (not impossible, remember—that is what good therapy is all about—but very difficult). Attachment theory is described in more detail in Chapter Sixteen.

It also has to do with recognizing boundaries and limits. For people with dissociative disorders, such recognition is so contrary to their experience of the world that it is almost ludicrous to expect it. After all, their boundaries and limits were never respected when they were young, so there was no way to have learned about such respect. The usual delicate recognition of a spouse's personal boundaries is one of the most difficult aspects of most close relationships, even if both partners have had an exemplary family life. Imagine what it must be like if one or—heaven forbid, but it happens—both partners are dissociative.

No wonder that in most families where there is a major dissociative disorder, including DDNOS (dissociative disorder not otherwise specified), family dysfunction is rife. Such dysfunction takes on many shapes and disguises: alcoholism or other addictions, behavior problems in the children, infidelity and/or other sexual problems (of either party or both parties), somatization, raging fights, school problems, work problems—the list often seems endless. When one also considers that the difficulties are being magnified both in content and context because of the varying personality characteristics of the different ego states in a highly dissociative DID, it is amazing that any kind of a positive relationship can be sustained.

It is particularly important to *watch the children* in such families very carefully. I'll speak about this in more detail in Chapter Fifteen, but vigilance on the part of the family physician is a must.

The beleaguered family doc will obviously wonder about counseling for this family, individually, as a couple, or as a group. Very, very seldom is it a good idea to attempt this yourself. For one thing, most of us are not trained to do this intense kind of family therapy; and, for another thing, the complexities of family counseling with dissociative disorders demands special training and experience. Even more important, perhaps, is the risk of alienating one parent or both, or the children. The parents, especially, will almost surely believe that you are taking sides, no matter how delicately you phrase your observations or suggestions. It's hard enough to do it in families where there are no dissociative disorders.

It is much wiser to search out counselors who are trained and experienced in the field. Your local chapter or association of psychologists, counselors, or (especially) marriage and family therapists can help you. And you can then maintain that support-ive role with the family which is so important to all concerned (even to you).

Anger-management problems present yet another challenge. They may occur in any of the family members, from different bases: in the nondissociative spouse, who begins to feel drowned in disorder and perceives him/herself to have completely lost control of his/her life; the dissociative spouse will without doubt have one raging ego state (the one who carries all the injustice of what happened during the childhood years) but this is seldom the part with whom you will be dealing because Rage usually stays in the background absorbing all the fury into him/herself and thus protecting the rest of the system. More often, it will be the ego state who is really angry but not raging who will go around smashing things or yelling; there may be one or more of the children who cannot deal with their feelings and so act out in a very belligerent way—usually this will disrupt the schoolyard and create havoc in the classroom.

Again, seek help from those who are trained in anger manage-ment (for yourself, too, so as to know how to respond if it erupts in one way or another in your consulting room) and present the suggestion of seeking counseling with great tact. You may find it useful to ask about the children's behavior at school and perhaps speak with the school counselor, but beware of confidentiality issues here.

You may find yourself in a tizzy with your colleagues. Professional relationships often take a real beating when your fellow GPs do not understand about dissociative disorders and wonder what in the world you are doing. This is one very good reason for you to stay completely away from the psychotherapy part of working with dissociation. You may find similar disruptions in your relationship with your psychiatric consultants. I have never really understood why, but many, if not most psychiatrists (at least in Canada and the U.S.) do not like to work with dissociative patients; for those referrals, we rely on our psychological colleagues. I was in the strange position of being an admitting member of the psychiatry department at our local hospital when I started working with Jayere—and subsequently with the others in my own family practice—and my relationship with that department, which had been great for fourteen years, was never the same again. Of course, it didn't help that I was flying by the seat of my pants because I had no idea, most of the time, how to handle the bizarre situations with which I was suddenly confronted. I truly believe that things are different now—but not as much as I would have hoped. Nevertheless, it's progress.

Be careful, then, to keep professional relationships clear of misunderstanding and be very upfront about discussing your situation *when* it is appropriate. A good presentation during rounds never hurts. Just get your references straight before you begin (see the research and reference material in Chapter Seventeen.)

Transference and countertransference are always with us, and never more so than in these challenging cases. Part of the problem lies in the comorbidity of dissociative patients—so often, they also fit the criteria for borderline personality disorder (the roots are the same, after all—a very dysfunctional family of origin) and it is usually the borderline characteristics that are so difficult to deal with.

It is not uncommon for the patient to perceive some similarity between the physician and some person the patient's own past, and that's where the transference comes in. Naturally, the patient is going to be suspicious (such patients have never earned to trust, remember) and start identifying you with that person. When you notice some apparent transference behavior, you may find it useful simply to mention it quietly, choosing both your words and the timing very carefully. You can be quite open; in fact, it is better if you are. "I'm wondering if there's something bothering you—perhaps something about me that reminds you of somebody else. Something I'm saying or doing. If so, let's talk about it."

That way, you ease the transference and usually abort the countertransference, and life becomes easier for everybody.

I spoke in the first paragraphs of this chapter about marital strife, and mentioned one husband who was very relieved when he and his wife were finally able to understand the dissociation. Sadly, though, it often happens that, with the best intention in the world, as the dissociative spouse works through his or her psychotherapy and begins to get better, the psychological and emotional strength of the spouse begins to deteriorate. I am sure that there are many reasons for this—plain old emotional fatigue might be one—but it sometimes happens that the nondissociative member of the marital relationship cannot cope with the changes that come through that same therapy. The wife (if it is she who is the patient) may start challenging his decisions, become more assertive, go out to work or quit a job she has decided she doesn't like, make new friends, attend social activities in which he is not included, or pursue some other course that is different from those she pursued before, both emotionally and behaviorally. He can't understand it, feels dislocated, and can't cope, and in time the marriage that was, ironically, held together by the need for the spouse to be strong and supportive falls apart when he is no longer needed in that role.

Of course, it is not only in close spousal relationships that one finds problems. Close friendships are equally difficult to establish and maintain. The social life of the dissociative patient is often very bleak indeed. In a different scenario, he or she may have an almost frantic social life but none of it is warm, nurturing, or reliable. It could (and often does) involve promiscuity or other somewhat dangerous pastimes. The trust issue comes up again— even the moderate amount of trust that we usually accord a good friend. The trust implicitly demanded in a very close friendship is often impossible. It is a recipe for depression and isolation, suspicious attitudes and a closing of doors that might otherwise lead to pleasant, rewarding relationships.

Such a life invites misunderstanding and leads to poor emotional health—which in turn can lead to poor psychophysiological health (remembering that we are never disconnected at the neck). Gentle inquiry into the patient's social functioning is as important as any other aspect of that person's health.

The same things could be said about relationships with others in the workplace. Of course, usually the patient has developed ego states whose specific job has to do with performing at work, so problems may not be so blatant. Coworkers may remark on a degree of moodiness or aloofness, often adding "... but she sure is a good worker!" For people who may not fully understand their own degree of dissociativity, these comments can be puzzling and upsetting. Our job as family physicians includes being alert to such factors, and inquiring about work satisfaction as a routine part of monitoring someone's health.

To reiterate:

- family dysfunction is rampant when there is a dissociative disorder
- it is important to watch the children for signs of behavior problems
- anger management may be very important
- arrange for trained colleagues to do any marital or family counseling
- recognize that one's own professional relationships may be affected
- understand transference and countertransference issues
- always be supportive, and discuss things openly but with tact
- social life and job satisfaction are important aspect of health.

Chapter Fifteen
For Children with Dissociative Parents

Of all the times we are the sentinels, surely our task in keeping children safe is the most important. This chapter is dedicated to those children whose mothers or fathers may be dissociative and—usually unwittingly—may put their children in jeopardy, physically or emotionally.

Secure attachments

All children deserve secure attachments—being able to know that there is at least one special person who will always be there for them and keep them safe. However, if your parent, especially your mother, is herself dissociative, it probably means that she has no idea how to do this.

I wrote briefly about attachment theory in the Introduction and Chapter Fourteen, and it is explained in even more detail in Chapter Sixteen. Basically, however, how well the "primary caretaker" (usually mother) can imbue that child with the essence of self-worth that means "my mother loves me and keeps me safe because I am special, I am *worthy*" is determined in large part by how secure her own sense of self-worth was similarly planted and nurtured when she herself was small. It's hard to teach something that you have never learned. That is why, in part, insecure attachments rank high in the transgenerational aspect of dissociative disorders.

Many, if not most, dissociative women have a well-developed "mother" ego state. They are committed to the role and very often execute it splendidly, even when other aspects of their personality structures are in chaos. Of course, we may quibble about what the mother believes to be "safe". For instance, I have a vivid memory of one of my dissociative patients who braved a main street in our community that had flood waters gushing down it from an over-flowing gully, carrying parts of trees and other chunky debris in its wake. She had the babe draped over her arm like a sack of potatoes because it was the day for baby's check-up and, of course, she was going to get to the doctor's office with that child, come hell or (literally) high water. I must say that babe was perfectly content to be so transported and grinned happily at me when the pair arrived in the office.

This chapter attends to some of the more common dangers for such children, and we need to watch carefully for clues as to their presence.

Unexplained injuries

Unexplained injuries in a young child, especially if that child appears repeatedly in the emergency room at the hospital or in the family physician's office with bruises, scrapes, burns (especially small, round, well-demarcated burns about the size of a cigarette end), broken bones or other evidence of trauma, deserve our immediate concern and attention. Often our first thought, especially if the child is very young, is battered-child syndrome, but it may be more complicated than that. For instance, although the child was injured at home by one of the parents, that parent may truly have no memory of perpetrating the abuse and be shocked when seeing the injuries—and even more shocked if she realizes that the doctor wonders if she did it. In fact, it had been another ego state, and there was a strong amnesia barrier between the two states.

And we have to remember that there may be another explanation. One of the items in a book I intend someday to write, entitled *Horrible Mistakes I Made When I Was Learning About Dissociation: All the Wrong Things to Do*, will be about the mother that both my nurse and I came to believe was abusing her child when actually it was the husband, and that poor woman was in constant fear of being beaten herself if she let on what was really happening. Many years later, when he was in jail, she was able to tell us how infuriated and helpless she felt when she realized that we hadn't believed her when she said she had not harmed the child. Had we looked more closely into her eyes, we might have been able to read some semblance of the truth.

Keeping children safe is the top priority. Most countries have laws about alerting the authorities if it is believed that a child is being abused. But herein lies another dilemma: if the parent truly doesn't remember doing anything bad, is she (or he) to be held responsible?

My answer is yes.

Perhaps that particular ego state doesn't remember, but some part of the system *does* know and it is vitally important for us to teach parents that such abuse must be stopped before it starts. It is a problem to be attended to closely in therapy, and our job is to make sure that it is recognized and properly handled.

Reluctance to divulge information

School counselors have often had the experience of recognizing that something is wrong with a child, but, when asked about it, the child hangs his head, muttering "I dunno" and scuffling his feet.

Children are immensely loyal and do not want to tell tales on their parents, no matter what the parents are doing. They are desperate to maintain the parents' love and refuse to talk about family fights, drunken dads (or moms), bullying big brothers, or other family "dysfunctions". Even gross physical or sexual abuse is covered up by children, who almost invariably believe that, if they are being abused, somehow they must have deserved it, it must be their fault. Young children are not capable of much abstract thought until the age of about eight years, and those megacognitive functions begin to evolve, and so everything that happens

129

must therefore be centered in themselves—there is no other way to comprehend it. And there is that subconscious need for secure attachment, which must never be ignored or jeopardized.

Such children deserve the attention of a counselor or psychologist who specializes in such matters and can use play therapy, for example, or role play, to elicit the truth. It is interesting that almost all children of dissociative parents take the fact of the different ego states for granted. (It's all they have known, remember.) They can tell you, if you win their confidence, about their various mothers: of the angry mother, or the Mommy who gets down on the floor and plays with them, or the Mommy who hugs Daddy and the one who doesn't. Children are not blind, and they are incredibly perceptive. But *telling* about bad or scary or painful things that happen—that's different.

Perfectionism

This is another common attribute of children with dissociative parents—the desperate need to be perfect.

For some, it might be an expression of, "If I can be better, maybe Mommy won't yell at me, or hit me, or Daddy won't do those things to me at night." Or, "If I get all perfect marks in school, then maybe that will make me a good girl and Daddy will love me more." The variations on the theme are endless.

I think the majority of children want to perform well, to be "good", so that their parents will express love and praise, but this kind of perfectionism goes well beyond that. It is similar to the need to be perfect that the anorexic suffers: "Maybe if I get thinner, I'll be a better person, just like my voices are telling me."

The school counselor, again, is often the best source of information about this state of affairs. Teachers pass along their concerns, and the child is invited in for a little chat, which is completely and adamantly not wanted by the child. However, sometimes the family doc can fulfill this role in a way that is more acceptable.

After all, doctors often ask questions about how someone is doing—it's normal. So we can be alert to such possibilities while not putting too much emphasis upon them.

Ask the youngster in your practice whom you know to be a child of a dissociative parent, or for whom you suspect this may be the case, casual questions about how school is going, whether she belongs to any teams or enjoys sports, what she likes best/least about school, whether she has a favorite teacher and, if so, what makes that teacher "favorite", and other similarly innocuous inquiries. If you have the good luck to have been that child's doctor literally since the day she was born, you'll not have any trouble chatting away on such matters and you may pick up on some interesting clues.

Behavior problems

Generally speaking, perfectionism seems to occur more in girls, and behavior problems seem more often to be seen in boys. I think this is a sort of cultural phenomenon: females attend to details, males attend to strong appearances. We have all met the opposite situations, of course.

Context may be important here. What is considered a behavior problem in one school may be virtually disregarded in another. Are there problems at home, too? Or in other settings besides school?

Bullying, bragging, inattention, talking out in class, strutting around, creating a sort of dissonance in the room, talking back and/or sassing the teacher or other adults, sending spitballs—you name it. All these attest to a great need to be heard and recognized for who you are, with the possible exception of bullying, which is in a different category and about which I'll write more a little further on.

Listen to how the parents describe these behaviors—if they seem to be distressed that their child is behaving in these ways, or whether they pass it off. Does it happen at home, too? If so, how is it handled, both by the dissociative and by the nondissociative parent? We can get a pretty good handle on the situation, and its relative importance, by asking a few questions, watching carefully for nonverbal communication, and listening. Are the parents comfortable with your querying the details? Are the children comfortable listening to their parents' answers?

We all know that children, with less vocabulary than adults by which to express their concerns or discomfort, resort to acting it out instead. In fact, we often call it "acting out". They will keep on with it, often getting more and more brazen, until they get the attention they need, and that means someone who will listen to them—*really* listen to them.

Bullying is in a different category. It expresses the need to dominate, to incite fear and trembling in the victim. Almost always it covers a great need to escape domination and/or scapegoating in their own lives. Virtually all bullies are being, or have also been, bullied. It is not uncommon for the father of a bully, for instance, to dismiss the problem as nonexistent or say something like, "The kid's just standing up for himself, just like I taught him. Good for him! No son of mine is going to grow up to be a wimp!" So the child expresses his fear by covering it up with bravado that goes beyond acceptable limits. I think the bully needs help desperately and it is imperative to get him or her into counseling with a good child psychologist.

Then, having done that, one pays attention to what is happening within the family that has been contributing to the behavior. Tact is required! But so is frank discussion. If you are lucky enough to be able to discuss these things with your patients (and of course, this applies to those families where there is a dissociative member and those where there is not a dissociative member), then you may be able to steer them in the right direction. It seems to me that, although children seem to take the bizarre case of having a variety of "mothers" in stride, it must also bring disquiet within their young minds, to say nothing of being teased by their friends. Children can be very cruel to each other. "Your mom's *sick*! She's *weird*! She's got *other people inside her*! Yuck!"

Faced with a barrage like that, what does the child do? Finds a way to fight back, of course.

When I hear that a child is having behavior problems, my immediate inner response is, "What's going on in that family?", because something is, and it needs to be expressed. It can be many things—a new sibling arrives, the pet rabbit dies, Dad has to go on business trips every week, Grandpa has come to live with us and he always gets drunk, some member of the family is ill or in the hospital, Grandma had a heart attack. If that "something" is a dissociative parent, we need to pay attention.

Another disturbing phenomenon is lying, especially when the child adamantly insists that she did *not* do what she is being accused of doing. "But I saw you do it," the teacher or parent or daycare worker might insist. "No, I *didn't do it!*"

One can usually tell if this denial is more than just wanting to get out of trouble, and that the child really seems to believe herself innocent. If that is your perception, from what you are told, then there is a much more worrisome possibility, and that is that the child is already becoming dissociative too. This means that action, the sooner the better, is needed.

Trouble making/keeping friends

Much of what has already been said about behavior also applies to the child who has trouble in making friends or, having made them, apparently discards them *or is discarded*, a short while later. When asked, "What happened to Bobby? You used to see so much of each other," one is answered with a shrug or a muttering under the breath.

This may be another example of kids' cruelty to each other. But there is another, more ominous possibility, and that is that the child is also becoming dissociative. Remember that dissociative disorders, especially those that are well along the spectrum, invariably have their roots in childhood. And also remember that many dissociative patients have one or more quite violent ego states.

We must never ignore this possibility, and, if you think you might recognize some symptoms—such as when the child seems to deny doing something that she has been seen to do—refer that child as soon as possible to a knowledgeable pediatric psychiatrist or psychologist who has the tools and experience to assess the situation. Dissociation in children is relatively easy to treat; the longer it goes on, the older the person becomes, the more complex the situation is likely to be. Act!

Urinary problems (congruent with age)

Dysuria, chronic urinary infections, eneuresis beyond normal age limits (i.e. after the age of ten), hematuria, vulvitis, vaginal discharge and other distress related to uncomfortable urinary, penile, or vulvovaginal function demands to be investigated in anybody, but even more imperatively with a child.

Of course one's mind immediately turns to abuse, and this must not be ruled out. If the child is very young, part of the difficulty may be in extracting the history, which is often dismissed as unimportant by the parent. This could be because the parent is the abuser, or because an ego state is the abuser unbeknown to other parts of the system, or because some other person—a friend or family member—is the perpetrator.

The problem may be quite different, of course, and be caused by other factors such as frequent and/or vigorous masturbation, but almost all children find their genitals and enjoy the sensations that go along with that, without acquiring any serious or ominous consequences.

Many children, however, intensely dislike any medical examination having to do with those sensitive parts of the body and put up quite a fuss about it. Fuss or no fuss, the cause must be found and appropriate treatment pursued. And that includes discovering how much the difficulty is related to a parent's, or other family member's, own dissociativity. Once the medical aspects are taken care of, family counseling might well be in order.

Unexplained abdominal pain

Virtually everything I have said about urinary problems applies to unexplained abdominal pain. Children do not normally have recurrent or chronic abdominal pain, so the appropriate investigations, again, are mandatory. This does not, however, mean that the child is subjected to ongoing investigations forever and ever. If "no reason" is found to account for the pain, then we are again back in the ream of "body memories", which can indeed occur in children.

Usually the source of the pain is one or both of two things: intense fear, e.g. of physical abuse, and sexual abuse.

Some children complain of abdominal pain (which I believe is real for them, as all pain is real to the person experiencing it) because they cannot face going to school. This may be because they are the victims of bullying or emotional abuse from their peers, or because they are inattentive in class and get into trouble from their teachers. Whatever the origin, the two aspects need attention: is there an organic cause for the pain; or is there fear, which is translated into pain?

As with other situations, if the child knows and trusts you, you may get further with the investigation than some stranger wearing a white coat, who wants to poke and prod and ask embarrassing questions. (Probably your colleague isn't like that at all, but that may be how the child perceives it.)

The only important thing is to make sure that the child is not in danger, physically or emotionally.

To sum up, when we have dissociative parents in our practices, it is imperative that we keep a vigilant eye on their children. Such children are very vulnerable and at risk for many different problems, including signals of becoming dissociative themselves. The sooner problems appear on the horizon, the more quickly they can be solved.

To reiterate:

- children being raised in a home with a dissociative parent are vulnerable
- watch for unexplained injuries, pain, or other symptoms that should not be present in healthy, happy children
- emotional problems, such as perfectionism or behavior disorders, may be caused by family dysfunction
- remember that children become dissociative too.

Chapter Sixteen
Neurophysiology

Over the past decade, the research into the neurophysiology of trauma and dissociation has positively erupted. Thanks to those wonderful people, the researchers, we are positively enlightened compared with what it was like fifteen or twenty years ago, regarding the ways in which stress, especially extreme and/or chronic stress, affects the brain and its functioning.

This has had a major impact on how we provide therapy, and some very important changes have been made. Many of those changes have to do with memory—that elusive phenomenon about which we have, in the past, been so mistaken.

I think it is useful to explain the basic pathways of mind–body connections to virtually all of our patients, and especially to those who have had trauma in their lives. My fairly simple and somewhat ingenuous way of doing so goes like this:

> An awareness, which is a kind of message, comes into our consciousness. That might be through sound, sight, smell, touch, taste—any and all of the senses provide us with those stimuli.

> The awareness passes through the layers of the conscious mind, neuron to neuron, and then continues its path as it reaches the levels of awareness we term "subconscious", still passing from neuron to neuron, brain cell to brain cell. Eventually, many of these messages reach a part of the brain known as the limbic system. The limbic system, a few clusters of cells deep within the right brain, is an extremely important part of our brains.

> Much more information awaits when the message reaches the limbic system. Previous messages, stored there, may add aspects that seem, to the brain, to be connected to the incoming stimulus. Memory and experience are stored in the limbic system; emotions are processed there; state-dependent learning (the emotional state we are in when we "learn"—i.e. experience—a situation and devise a way to respond to it predicates how we will probably

respond when a similar type of experience comes our way again) is to be found in the limbic system; probably altered states of consciousness—meditation, hypnosis, perhaps deep prayer—rely on the limbic system for processing. All of this previous information modifies the incoming message, as do psychosocial factors and environmental input.

This modified message now continues on its way, down the part of the brain known as the *hypothalamus*. The hypothalamus can be thought of as the most deeply knowledgeable part of the brain, in the sense that it is really the most basic source of experiential knowledge. It then passes, through biochemical messengers now, across to the pituitary gland. The pathway by which that journey that I have just described is followed is known as the *limbic–hypothalamic–pituitary axis*.

The pituitary is the granddaddy gland in the body. Its hormones affect and regulate all the other endocrine glands—those that secrete hormones—in the body. It sends out the hormones to those glands that, it its wisdom, the pituitary thinks are most involved with this evolving situation.

Those glands—for example, the adrenals or the reproduction glands or the thyroid gland—respond to this stimulus from the pituitary by sending out their own hormones, and the various organs in the body respond accordingly. The heart beats faster, the sexual organs are excited, the thyroid sends out more thyroxin—whichever action is prompted by the message from the pituitary.

And then the body sends its own response back to the limbic system! It is the quintessential biofeedback mechanism. That return information may stay there, adding to the resident information in that tiny but crucial part of the brain, or it may continue its journey back to the conscious mind and we become aware of some kind of response.

Well, I told you that it was ingenuous.

The basic conceptualization, however, is very important and this description comes, somewhat modified, from Ernest Rossi's wonderful book, *The Psychobiology of Mind–Body Healing* (1986). I have explained it, in just this way, to almost every patient who has had some trauma—emotional, physical, or sexual—in his or her life; none have found it hard to understand, and all have found it to be, in some way, comforting. It *explains* things. It helps them to know that there is a reason for their feeling and responding the way they have been doing.

Of course, the discourse above has to do with those awarenesses that come into conscious perception in some way; it says nothing about the implicit, experiential knowledge, which is far more common and also has far more impact.

Stress and the brain

Figure 16.1: Stress and the brain

- Extreme stress "shuts down" the thinking brain, especially the language areas of the left hemisphere.

- This "short circuits" the cognitive system, leaving only the autonomic reactions of the stress response.

STRESS	DEFENSE MECHANISM
Freeze	*Dissociate*
	Projection, Displacement
Flee	Denial, Rationalization
	Distortion etc.
Fight	

- Powerful emotions, generated in the **right hemisphere**, cannot be processed in the **left** (no language).

- Stress (chronic, severe) inhibits the flow of information **within** the brain, and between brain and body.

Extreme stress "shuts down" the brain, especially the language areas of the left hemisphere. This short-circuits the cognitive system, leaving only the autonomic reactions of the stress response. Because of this shutdown, all those powerful, overwhelming emotions that the trauma has generated in the right hemisphere—the *experiential* hemisphere, if you will—cannot be processed in the left language-and-logic part of the brain. Have you ever heard somebody say, "There are no words to express how I feel"? It can be literally true, and in such a situation the emotions that cannot be expressed in words continue to be expressed in feelings, churning and ever more churning around in the right limbic system. I think of it as a kind of emotional abscess, and abscesses, as you know, cannot heal until they are opened, drained, and cleaned out. *Then* they heal.

And so we help them to put it into words by listening, being there, making helpful noises and "bearing witness". That's what psychotherapy is all about.

Of course, as a family physician you may feel that this is probably not your role most of the time, although occasionally it may be. You can help, however, by explaining that emotions and logic have nothing whatever to do with each other (if emotions were logical they wouldn't be emotions); that you know your patient is not crazy; and that going to someone who understands about trauma and its impact might be helpful.

Extreme stress, therefore, inhibits the flow of information both within the brain and between brain and body. Nevertheless, it has to be expressed somehow, and thus the plethora of otherwise unexplainable symptoms evolves.

Remember that the brain is designed to adjust its chemistry and electrical circuitry to meet the demands of the environment, internal and external. Experience determines which circuits or neuronal loops will become activated and joined together (sort of a "use it or lose it" situation). As always, circuits that are repeatedly activated, *positively or negatively*, are strengthened and stabilized and they can therefore be turned on with less and less stimulation, which accounts for the fact that, in time, people with post- traumatic stress disorder respond with overwhelming distress to what most of us would think of as a minor event. Furthermore, and this is the scary part, normal response seems to have been changed *forever* as the brain responds to the now negatively adjusted, post-traumatic chemistry of the adrenergic system.

Figure 16.2: Sensitization: use-dependent development

- The brain is designed to adjust its chemistry and electrical circuitry to meet the needs of the environment.

- Experience determines which circuits of neurons become activated and join together.

- Circuits that are repeatedly activated (**positively or negatively**) are strengthened and stabilized, and can be turned on with less and less stimulation (**positive or negative**).

- Parts of the brain mature at different ages and stages of the person—how those parts work together depends on the experiences to which the child is exposed (**positive or negative**).

I must add that there is new research information that ameliorates this desolate conclusion somewhat (see Rossi, 2002). Over the decades, continuing attention has been given to war veterans who have shown decreases in hippocampal size. Just in the past few years, there is now a suggestion that, in some, the hippocampus seems to be increasing in volume again. The term used is *neurogenesis* and it implies that brain cells can, indeed, regenerate. It has to do with what is being called "gene expression". This is totally against what I was taught in medical school! But it is very exciting.

Parts of the brain mature at different ages and stages; how those parts work together depends on the experience to which the child is exposed, positive or negative. Put this into the context of traumatized children and we can understand a little better how their coping skills as adults are often dismally ineffective, if not outright sabotaging. In response to a question I posed at a lecture I attended a year or so ago, regarding the effects of chronic, severe emotional abuse to a child of four years of age, Dr John McArdle responded that it would be like hitting her in the head with a baseball bat, severely impairing the child's ability to devise new, appropriate coping skills as she grew up, and consequently always, apparently, responding in a very childish way. Dr McArdle is a well-respected international authority on intellect and intelligence.

In fact, this is not really a new understanding at all. Charcot and Janet, in Europe, and William James, in the U.S. recognized more than a hundred years ago: "… on the one hand, the flexibility of the mind and on the other, how certain memories become obstacles that kept people from going on with their lives" (van der Kolk and van der Hart, 1991, page 425). One wonders why these simple yet elegant appreciations of how the mind works were dismissed for so long.

Memory

And this brings us to memory. As we now know, there are two very different kinds of memory. One is called *implicit* memory. It is present when we are born—indeed, perhaps before we are born, which gives some credence to the claim that people can remember what it was like when they were in the womb. Think of that agitated newborn, put up on its mother's chest. It settles right down, listening to the heartbeat that it remembers so well.

Implicit memory is behavioral, perceptual, emotional, somatosensory memory. It is probably the source of what are called "body memories", that so many trauma-spectrum patients describe. It is also probably the link between the pain of fibromyalgia, for example, and the trauma that so many of those who have this diagnosis also have experienced.

We don't have to pay attention for this type of memory to be stored in our memory banks—those memory banks that are located in the limbic system. It just happens, and one is then stuck with the memories, unprocessed, until they are expurgated through psychotherapy of one sort or another.

Attachment experiences, which I will discuss in more detail later, also become stored (the term used is *encoded*) in the same memory banks.

Figure 16.3

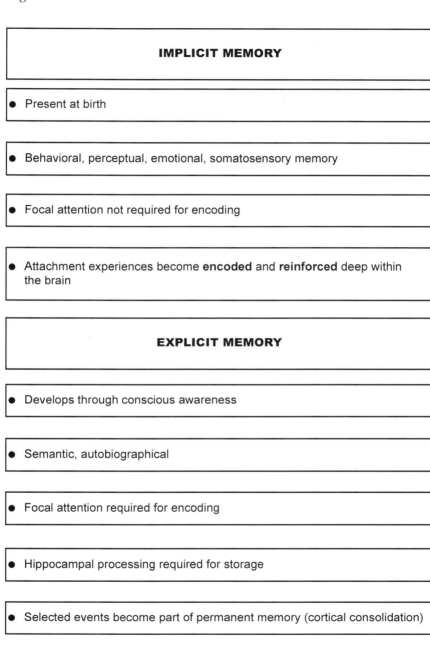

IMPLICIT MEMORY

- Present at birth

- Behavioral, perceptual, emotional, somatosensory memory

- Focal attention not required for encoding

- Attachment experiences become **encoded** and **reinforced** deep within the brain

EXPLICIT MEMORY

- Develops through conscious awareness

- Semantic, autobiographical

- Focal attention required for encoding

- Hippocampal processing required for storage

- Selected events become part of permanent memory (cortical consolidation)

- **Narrative** memory

Explicit memory is quite different, because it develops through conscious awareness. It is autobiographical, that is to say memory that can be described in words. "I remember when …" we often say, and we are then referring to explicit memories. Many of these memories are laced with emotion—good, bad, happy, sad—but they have been processed through the hippocampus and transferred, as it were, to a different shelf in the library.

We do have to pay attention for these kinds of memory to be encoded. (If we had not, we would never have passed those exams in medical school.) The brain, utilizing the talents of the hippocampus, then stores selected events and experiences and knowledge as part of permanent memory, a process known as *cortical consolidation*. Such memory involves megacognitive function and therefore is associated with the developing brain as it matures. Most of us find that memories are more clearly recalled when the experiences occurred as we got older, through kindergarten into school, and thus we began to create a narrative of our lives.

The big exception, of course, is memory related to trauma, which is experiential and therefore implicit, but breaks through to hand us a double whammy at the most unexpected times, having been triggered by some small reminder that consciously we don't even recognize half the time.

Van der Kolk and van der Hart remind us (1991) that Janet described healthy psychological functioning as dependent upon the unified memory of all segments of the experience—emotions, thoughts, actions, sensations: in other words, the BASK (behavior, affect, sensation, knowledge) model described by Braun in 1986.

I have spoken before about all memory as being malleable. This is because memories are constantly being reworked, like a piece of clay in the hands of a sculptor. Why then do some memories seem to get "fixed" in the mind and resistant to change from subsequent experiences? Van der Kolk and van der Hart suggest that this may occur though myelinization. Remembering that the brain develops at different ages and stages, it is the myelinization process that "fixes" memories (1991, page 442).

Where does psychotherapy fit into this pattern of events? It seems that one must return to the old memory often in order to complete it, to unify the fragments. Nobody likes doing this very much, in the case of memories of abuse or trauma, yet it is exactly those experiences that most need to be processed and finally put to rest on the cognitive shelf in that internal library where they will cease to intrude, having been divested of so much of their psychological and emotional reactions.

Where do dissociation and chronic syndromes overlap in all of this? Scaer (2001) remarks that explicit memory, which involves the hippocampus and other prefrontal cortical pathways, is notoriously vulnerable to "decay", i.e. the memory disintegrates over time and reinvents itself in a slightly changed pattern. We need to remember this when we are listening to patients recall traumatic events. On the other hand, implicit memories, especially if they swirl around threats and emotional upheaval, are very resistant to decay and this, Scaer believes, is the extremely strong, virtually unbreakable link, a conditioned response, that keeps the neural loops of trauma and dissociation activated.

The neural pathways involved in these links and the perpetuation of them, seem to involve mainly the locus ceruleus, amygdala, thalamus, hippocampus, and right orbitofrontal cortex, as van der Kolk described in his epic paper, "The Body Keeps the Score" (1994). He goes on to say that people who actively dissociate during traumatic events are more likely to develop PTSD symptoms that those who do not. Children, of course, are very vulnerable and almost always dissociate during trauma.

Somatic dissociation—the apparent splitting off of perceptions in parts of the body and creating those irritating complaints (irritating to the physician—other words might more justly describe the feelings of the patient) that seem to have no anatomical explanation, such as stocking and glove anesthesia—is not well addressed in medical literature. They are usually dismissed as conversion disorders, a diagnostic technique that infuriates the patient. Chronic syndromes such as fibromyalgia or chronic fatigue syndromes are sometimes also lumped into these categories. Personally, I prefer the concept of the body's reminding us that old traumas are not forgotten, they just keep on being expressed in a different way.

Much of the PTSD response is the "freeze" part of the flight-or-fight process. Freeze always comes first, and then comes the flight or fight. But what if you can neither flee nor fight (which applies to most children)? You dissociate. This sets up, Scaer and others believe, a cycle of dysregulation in the autonomic system, having to do basically with parasympathetic response. The so-called "chronic diseases of unknown cause" are prime examples of this type of dysregulation, and of the suffering that accompanies it.

Attachment

Attachment theory has now become one of the most explored aspects of why some people are so vulnerable and others are not.

All living things, especially young living things, have a need to feel securely connected to a protective source. I see the tiny duck-lings in the park near where I live, as mother duck squawks at them and hustles them under her breast feathers (which then puff out like a formidable dowager) if one of the local herons is looking on with too much interest. Or think of any creature in the animal kingdom, looking out for its young. Think, too, of pods of whales, dolphins, and other sea mammals, which offer safety for each other. It's not so hard to believe that humans need these connections, too.

I have already referred two or three times to attachment theory. I don't apologize for doing so again, because I believe that it is so important.

About 35 years ago, Bowlby (1969) described his recognition of three distinctly different ways in which very young children responded to their primary caregiver, usually the mother. Everybody thought it was interesting, but then it was almost for-gotten until Mary Ainsworth, decided to explore it in much more depth a decade later. The result was a work called the "Strange Situation", which was published in 1978.

This work proved the patterns described by Bowlby. Furthermore, it became the root of a magnificent piece of sociological research, which in time involved universities in several countries and provided many thousands of case histories.

Later, Judith Solomon and Mary Main joined in the research; in 1986 they described a fourth pattern, Disorganized/Disoriented, and Main and Morgan linked this type of infant response to dissociative states in their 1996 paper (see Chapter Seventeen).

In essence, the four attachment patterns were described as *secure*, *ambivalent*, *avoidant*, and *disorganized*. When the mothers were asked to describe what it was like when *they* were growing up, their answers reflected the same kinds of pattern. As I tell my patients (to help them to understand that we are not blaming the mother, but just discovering how some problems may have originated) that it is very hard to teach what you have never learned.

Let me make this very clear: this is not an excuse for abuse, but simply offers some insight about the perpetrator. Often, though, Mother is not the perpetrator, but neither is she able to step in and protect the child. She has never learned how, nor has she had a role model to follow.

Lucky children who have had secure attachments are much more resilient to the vagaries of life as they grow up. They know how to trust, and how to differentiate when trusting is not the thing to do. If they are endangered in any way, including emotionally, they have better coping skills.

However, if one is not sure about trusting, or avoids the whole concept and just wishes it would go away, or simply dissolves or explodes into disorganization, that person becomes very vulnerable indeed should trauma come into his life. As we remember the terrible PTSD of the Vietnam veterans, all the research supports the fact that those most affected had come from very dysfunctional homes.

Attachment, or lack of it, is therefore an important factor in all the trauma-spectrum disorders, and recognizing its importance helps us to unravel some of the astonishing responses that we see in our dissociative and/or chronic patients. You can imagine, for example, that highly dissociative patients might have developed one protector or more in their internal systems, to compensate for what was missing in their early childhood experiences. Indeed, it might be such a protector who takes you to task if she feels that you are not doing your job properly. Curb your counter-transference and recognize the truly remarkable—almost Herculean—job that the patient has done to compensate for what was never available to him when it should have been, to fill in the gaps of memory, to provide some semblance of continuity in a discontinuous conscious awareness despite the evolution of those difficult and intrusive neurological pathways and memory constructs.

Putting all of this into context of trauma and the brain, we have some key points:

- Mental capacities are *developmental* achievements, depending on the maturation of the orbitofrontal and other areas of the prefrontal cortex.
- Development of the orbitofrontal cortex depends on the strength of secure attachments in very early childhood.
- Chronic stress/trauma inhibits the processing of experience and memory from the implicit (right-brain, limbic system) to the explicit (left-brain, language and logic system) through the hippocampus.
- Repeated activation of neuronal patterns (sensitization) strengthens those patterns, positively *or* negatively.
- The hippocampus in individuals who have suffered extreme, ongoing trauma, is smaller than normal.
- Psychological/emotional effects of trauma are stored in somatic (implicit) memory.
- In psychotherapy, traumatic memories can gradually be put into words ("creating the narrative").
- It is now thought that, through processes known as neurogenesis and *gene expression*, hippocampal activity can improve and the hippocampus itself can increase in size, toward normal volume. This occurs, for example, in psychotherapy, where the

implicit memories of the trauma are processed, the narrative created, and the memory introduced into the left-brain, explicit memory bank.

Through understanding some of the neurological aspects, we are better able to put our experiences with dissociative and chronic patients into context.

Chapter Seventeen
Research and References

In this chapter you will find the references for all the articles and books specifically mentioned throughout the book, as well as some other references which you may find interesting. I have arranged it according to chapter.

Introduction

Bowlby, J. (1969), *Attachment and Loss,* Vol. I, *Attachment* (New York, NY: Basic Books).

Braun, Bennett (1986), *Treatment of Multiple Personality Disorder* (Washington, D.C.: American Psychiatric Press).

Braun introduced the concept of the BASK model. If one is to help people piece together fragmented memories, then the understanding that the aspects of *be*havior, *a*ffect, *s*ensation and *k*nowledge (cognition) must all be united to form a cohesive whole is crucial. Various parts of the personality structure carry this knowledge and the information that those parts of the system hold is retrieved by the patient as the memory unfolds. It is *very* important that patients discover these aspects themselves, without our input or interpretations. We gently guide them to find their own truths, rather than tell them what those truths "should" be.

Braun was one of the founding fathers of the International Society for the Study of Multiple Personality and Dissociation (now known as the International Society for the Study of Dissociation).

Putnam, F. W. (1989), *Diagnosis and Treatment of Multiple Personality Disorder* (New York, NY: Guilford Press).

Putnam, with his colleague Dr. Eva Carlson, devised one of the first diagnostic questionnaires for use with those who may have dissociative disorders, the Dissociative Experiences Scale. After twenty years, it is still one of the most useful tools for those who are interested in sorting out the differential diagnosis of many patients whose symptoms are particularly puzzling. More recently, there has been an modification that many therapists find useful, a "taxon" version, which identifies those situations more likely to indicate a disorder, compared with the others—much more common—that really simply indicate a capacity for dissociative experience.

Schafer, Donald: Schafer is a psychiatrist in California who has been interested in this field for many years. His comments to me, when I was wondering what on earth to do about this interesting but confusing new patient whom I had acquired from my friend and colleague, were what really started me on this journey into the hearts and minds of those who have been traumatized. Although there have been days when I wished I'd never heard of dissociation, it has been (and continues to be) the basis of some of the most fascinating journeys I have ever taken with my patients—learning from them and utterly admiring their tenacity to get well.

Siegel, Daniel (1999), *The Developing Brain: Toward a neurolobiology of interpersonal experience* (New York, NY: Guilford Press).

This excellent book, which discusses memory, attachment, emotion, self-regulation and many other aspects of the psyche, is easy to read and full of insights. You may want it on your bookshelf—I recommend it as a book every physician should read.

Watkins J. G. and Watkins H. H. (1992), *Hypnosis and Ego State Therapy: Innovations in clinical hypnosis: A source book*, Vol. 10 (Sarasota, FL: Professional Resource Exchange), pp. 23–27.

Dr. Jack Watkins and his wife Helen Watkins were in the forefront of therapeutic approaches for working with dissociative patients. Their specialty was the concept of Ego State Therapy, about which they have written several books and many articles.

Chapter One

Hunter, M. E. (2002), "Degree of Dissociativity in the Street Population in Victoria, British Columbia", research paper presented at the conference on "Making the Connections", University of Victoria, May.

This paper compiled questionnaires given to twenty "street people"—all young and apparently healthy. They all had enough get-up-and-go to enlist in a training course for job applications, and learned two trades: the basics of the fast-food industry and janitorial skills. The success rate of this particular project was extremely high—about 86 percent. They also learned coping skills, self-esteem, and other life strategies.

Eighteen of the twenty had significant dissociative characteristics. And these were those who were able to get themselves into the project: how about all those who were unable to get that far?

Nijenhuis, E. (1999), *Somatoform Dissociation* (Assen, The Netherlands: van Gorcum and Co.), see Chapter Seven.

Chapter Three

Birnbaum, M. H. and Thomann, K. (1996), "Visual function in MPD", *Journal of the American Optometric Association*, Vol. 67 (6), pp. 327–34.

I confess that I have not actually read this article. There is a large amount of anecdotal evidence that various DID alters have differing visual capacity: some need glasses, others don't some are color blind, others aren't. I have included the reference thinking that perhaps it might intrigue you.

Hunter, M. E. (1986), "Variable thyroid hormone results in multiple personality alters", paper presented at the Fourth International Conference on Multiple Personality and Dissociation, Chicago.

Miller, S. D. and Triggiano, P. J. (1992), "A psychophysiological investigation of multiple personality disorder: Review and update", *American Journal of Clinical Hypnosis*, Vol. 35 (1) pp. 47–61.

The authors presented the first comprehensive review of the neurophysiology of dissociative disorders up to that time. Although there has been a great deal of research since then, this paper was nevertheless a landmark in the literature.

Tsai, G. E., Condie, D., Wu, M. T. and Chang, I. V. V., (1999), "Functional MRI of personality switching", *Harvard Review of Psychiatry*, July–August, Vol. 7 (2), pp. 119–22.

This article focuses on the changes in functional MRI between DID ego states, adding to the neurological understanding of this disorder.

Chapter Five

Bjerklund-Johansen, T. E. and Weider, J. (2002). "Current Opinions in Urology", Vol. 12 (1), pp. 63–67.

The authors undertook this study because there had been nothing, previously, in the literature as to objective findings, particularly in the case of male chronic pelvic-pain syndromes.

However, new research on an inflammatory response in expressed prostatic secretion (in patients with this syndrome) and in bladder tissue samples from patients with interstitial cystitis have the researchers wondering about cytokine gene expression and what is going on in those complex areas. They are also very interested in new drugs that relieve the inflammatory response in these conditions.

Cohen, H., et al. (2002), "Prevalence of post-traumatic stress disorder in fibromyalgia patients: overlapping syndromes or post-traumatic fibromyalgia syndrome?", *Seminars in Arthritis and Rheumatology*, Vol. 32 (1) pp. 38–50.

This was the first comprehensive study that applied structural clinical assessment of trauma exposure and PTSD in fibromyalgia patients. The study showed a significant overlap in PTSD symptoms and fibromyalgia symptoms (according to the diagnostic criteria for each).

It has been known for some time that the incidence of a history of child abuse and dysfunctional families is significantly higher in fibromyalgia patients. This study confirms the impressive statistical overlap of these two syndromes.

Crawford, H. (1995), "Brain dynamic shifts during hypnotic analgesia: Why can't we all eliminate pain?", American Society of Clinical Hypnosis, Chicago.

In this invited plenary address, Crawford discussed the possibility that some people become supersensitized to pain at the central level. She suggested that such a scenario might be as follows: the person is involved in an accident or severe physical abuse; he or she recovers; then, at a later date, there is another incident; although the second incident does not seem very severe in itself, the brain overreacts and the smallest sensation—a finger gently stroking the arm, for example—is perceived as being severe pain.

Crawford H. H., et al. (1998), "Hypnotic analgesia: I. Somato-sensory event-related potential changes to noxious stimuli, and II.

Transfer learning to reduce chronic low back pain", *International Journal of Clinical and Experimental Hypnosis*, Vol. 46, pp. 92–132.

Gerdle, B. (2002), "Are perceived muscle tension, electromyographic hyperactivity and personality traits correlated in the fibromyalgia syndrome?", *Journal of Rehabilitation Medicine*, Vol. 34, (2) pp. 73–80.

The author and his colleagues found that neither perceived muscle tension nor "muscular tension personality trait" correlated with EMG hyperactivity. However, perceived general muscle tension did correlate with aspects of anxiety-proneness. The suggestion from the author, therefore, is that, when patients with fibromyalgia report muscle tension, they may actually be expressing some other factor, such as anxiety, rather than physiological tension.

Hunter, M. E. (1994), *Making Peace with Chronic Pain: A Whole-Life Strategy* (New York, NY: Brunner/Mazel).

This book offers an ego-state approach to the problem of chronic pain syndromes, in the form of a metaphor of the Dance. Of course, it is just one of many approaches but at times its comparative novelty opens doors for some patients to perceive their pain syndrome differently, and therefore offers some new opportunity for relieving the intrusion of pain into their lives.

Jerome, J. (1993), "Transmission or transformation? Information processing theory of chronic human pain", *APS Bulletin* 2(3): pp. 160–71.

Jerome suggests that the suffering associated with chronic pain is due, at least in part, to a breakdown or alteration of the information processing at a central brain level, resulting in an inability to process and integrate additional incoming data. This in turn results in a deficit in the ability to devise and/or elicit good effective coping strategies.

He therefore presents a flow chart, indicating the sequence of events that results in a reinforcing of the perception and memory of pain.

Lee, J. C., Yang, C. C., Kromm, B. G. and Berger, R. E. (2001), "Neurophysiologic testing in chronic pelvic-pain syndrome: A pilot study", *Urology*, Vol. 58 (2), pp. 246–50.

Because studies of male chronic pelvic-pain syndrome have generally focused on prostate pathology rather than on the neurology of pain, the authors decided to research small, unmyelinated C fibers that mediate heat and visceral pain rather than the integrity of somatosensory nerve pathways consisting of large "Group A Fibers". They hypothesized that chronic pelvic-pain syndrome was mediated through these small fibers. The results showed that the large myelinated fibers do not play a significant role in the pathophysiology of chronic pelvic-pain syndrome: rather, there is an altered sensation of perineal pain elicited by heat, which may represent a C-fiber-mediated effect.

Lidbeck, J. (2002), "Central hyperexcitability in chronic musculoskeletal pain: A conceptual breakthrough with multiple clinical applications", *Pain Research and Management*, Vol. 7 (2), pp. 81–92.

The author points out that the growing awareness and acceptance of dysfunctional central pain modulation may be what he terms a conceptual breakthrough leading to better understanding of such disorders.

Lumley, M. A., Smith, J. A. and Longo, D. J. (2002), "The relationship of alexithymia to pain severity and impairment among patients with chronic myofascial pain: comparisons with self-efficacy, catastrophizing, and depression", *Journal of Psychosomatic Research*, Vol. 53 (3), pp. 823–30.

The authors point out that alexithymia is elevated in chronic pain patients, but its relationship to the severity of the pain is not clear.

Although it would seem that the alexithymia is not related to the sensory component of pain, it does correlate positively with the affective or unpleasant component of pain—in other words, the suffering component. It is also related positively to catastrophizing and a sense of self-reliance.

Melzack, R. (1990), "Phantom limbs and the concept of a neuromatrix", *Trends in Neuroscience*, Vol. 13 (3), pp. 88–92.

Melzack is best known for the "Gate" explanation of pain. He is constantly looking toward better theories to explain how and why people respond to pain in such variable ways. His neuromatrix and "neurosignature" approach is one of many possible explanations that this inventive and open-minded theorist explores.

Smith, J. A., Lumley, M. A. and Longo, D. J. (2002), "Contrasting emotional approach coping with passive coping for chronic myofascial pain", *Annals of Behavioral Medicine*, Vol. 24 (4), pp. 326–35.

Although emotional approach coping (EAC) has been studied in some nonpain populations, it had not been studied in a chronic-pain population. The results would indicate that EAC could be a useful approach, as it was related to less affective pain and less depression. The study points out the need to assess emotional coping processes that are not confused or impacted by distress or dysfunction.

Wikner J., Hirsch, U., Wetterberg, L. and Rojdmark, S. (1998), "Fibromyalgia—a syndrome associated with decreased nocturnal melatonin secretion", *Clinical Endocrinology*, Vol. 49 (2) p. 179 ff.

This finding is particularly interesting in light of the fact that sleep disturbances pay such a role in the chronic syndromes that we have studied. Perhaps adding melatonin to the pharmacological treatment of fibromyalgia patients could be helpful.

Zermann, D. H., Ishigooka, M., Doggweiler-Wiygul, R., Schubert, J. and Schmidt, R. A. (2001), "The male chronic pelvic pain syndrome", *World Journal of Urology*, Vol. 19 (3); pp. 173–79.

These authors also are looking toward a neurobehavioral perspective to explain the pathways and neurophysiological mechanisms for male chronic pelvic-pain syndrome, and thence to divide treatment into causal and symptomatic approaches.

Chapter Six

Abbey, Susan: Dr. Susan Abbey is a highly respected member of the psychiatric community in Canada. At present she is the President of the Canadian Psychiatric Association.

Natelson, B. H. and Lange, G. (2002), "A status report on chronic fatigue syndrome", *Environmental Health Perspectives Supplements*, Vol. 110 (4), pp. 673–78.

The overview of the current status of chronic fatigue syndrome once again concludes by saying that there are still no medical explanations. However, they say, there are several possible pathophysiological processes: a covert encephalopathy, impaired physiological capability to respond to physical and mental stressors, and the possibility that effort exacerbates symptoms, all of which are under ongoing investigation.

Pols, R. (2003), "Somatisation of psychological problems. ('Who Cares?') Connection", August, paper presented at the Inaugural Scientific Conference in Australia.

Pols described a model of somatization disorder especially useful for the general practitioner. He links a predisposition, a critical incident that activates assumptions, leading to affective symptoms and cognitions with a somatic focus, all of which then aggravate the disorder and further engrain the cycle.

He suggests that vulnerable patients then get better and better at detecting symptoms, and "recruitment" of other symptoms follows.

Sabath, D. E., Barcy, S., Koelle, D. N., Zeh, J., Ashton, S. and Buchwald, D. (2002), "Cellular immunity in monozygotic twins discordant for chronic fatigue syndrome", *Journal of Infectious Diseases*, Vol. 185 (6), pp. 828–31.

Twin studies have an inherent validity that no other studies can have: exactly the same genetic background. Therefore, disparate genetic factors can be ruled out when assessing for interference in the protocol of the study. This article was designed to assess immune function in patients suffering from chronic fatigue syndrome by assessing lymphocyte cell surface markers and NK activity. Significantly greater variability was noted in the twins discordant for CFS than in concordant healthy twins. The authors stress the need for further studies.

Sullivan, M. and Katon, W. (1993), "Somatization: The path between distress and somatic symptoms", *APS Bulletin*, Vol. 2 (3), pp. 141–49.

The authors describe the process by which somatic symptoms are reinforced and cause the maintenance rather than the diminishing of the somatization. They feel that modification of physician behavior is crucial to this process.

It is an excellent article on the types and process of somatization and the perspective, in their view, of primary care, and makes a plea for much better information sharing among physicians, psychologists, and physiologists.

Other articles and reports on CFS can be found on the Internet.

Chapter Seven

Bowman, E. (1993), "Etiology and clinical course of pseudo-seizures. Relationship to trauma, depression and dissociation." *Psychosomatics*, Vol. 34, pp. 333–42.

Bowman was a pioneer in the study of pseudoseizures and especially with their possible link to dissociative experience. Four psychodynamic pathways to such pseudoseizures were noted: most commonly, they were linked to separate ego states, being expressions of dissociated memories of child abuse, and had been triggered by some recent stress or trauma.

Drossman, D. A. and Thompson, W. G. (1992), "The irritable bowel syndrome: Review and a graduated multicomponent approach", *Annals of Internal Medicine*, Vol. 116 (12) (Part 1), pp. 1009–16.

The authors considered the epidemiology, pathophysiology, and psychosocial factors while devising a conceptual model to answer the question "Why is the patient coming in now?" Treatment approaches for mild, moderate, and severe cases are presented.

Farthing, M. J. G. (1995), "Irritable bowel, irritable body or irritable brain?", *British Medical Journal*, Vol. 310, January, pp. 171–75.

This article challenges the concept that the problem is one of bowel function and motility, questioning instead the role of other psychological factors. The author maintains that increased visceral sensation in patients with this syndrome may be a crucial factor in the disorder. It is a well-organized and thought-provoking article, which offers a psychosomatic model for the condition.

Francis, C. Y. and Houghton, L. A. (1996), "Use of hypnotherapy in gastrointestinal disorders", *European Journal of Gastroenterology and Hepatology*, Vol. 8 (6), pp. 525–29.

This is an overview article of the areas of gastrointestinal disorders in which hypnotherapy has been used; particular attention has been paid to irritable bowel syndrome.

The main problem has been that most reports have been anecdotal. Nevertheless, patients are reported to have benefited from the approach.

Goldberg, J. and Davidson, P. (1997), "A biopsychosocial understanding of the irritable bowel syndrome: A Review", *Canadian Journal of Psychiatry*, Vol. 42 (8), pp. 835–40.

This is a review article of the literature about irritable bowel syndromes. The results indicated that the condition is very common, but few patients actually seek help and, if they do, are usually reassured by simple explanations and target symptom-directed treatment. An exception is with those patients who seek psychiatric help, who generally have not experienced relief through the more simple techniques. However, this small group consume considerable healthcare resources.

Gomborone J., Dewsnap, P., Libby, G. and Farthing, M. (1995), "Abnormal illness attitudes in patients with irritable bowel syndrome", *Journal of Psychosomatic Research*, Vol. 39 (2), pp. 227–30.

As one can tell from the title, this paper discusses what the authors describe as the psychosocial dimension of illness behavior. Dimensions are provided by the illness attitude scales, which discriminate sensitively between patients with hypochondriasis and those without.

It is an interesting paper and sure to arouse some angst in the hearts of those who may perceive it as somewhat dismissive of the reality—for the patient—of his or her symptoms.

Griffith, J. L., Polles, A. and Griffith, M. E. (1998), "Pseudoseizures, Families and Unspeakable Dilemmas", *Psychosomatics*, Vol. 39, pp. 144–53.

The authors studied patients with pseudoseizures and their families to discover what relationship, if any, the pseudoseizures have to family distress. The result, as predicted, indicated an "unspeakable dilemma", which it was very difficult for the family to discuss, in almost all cases.

Houghton, L. A., Heyman, D. J. and Whorwell, P. J. (1996), "Symptomatology, quality of life, and economic features of irritable bowel syndrome—the effects of hypnotherapy", *Alimentary Pharmacology and Therapeutics*, Vol. 10 (1), pp. 93–95.

Whorwell is known as the pioneer in the use of hypnosis to relieve the symptoms of irritable bowel syndrome. In this article he and his colleagues wanted to quantify the effects of this approach on quality of life and economic functioning.

The study showed unequivocal benefits through improvements to the patients' quality of life and reduces work absenteeism.

Landau, M. (2001), "Conversion disorders", *www.eMedicine.com*.

I discovered this article on the Internet while searching for pseudocoma. It is one of the few references to pseudocoma that I found, but it does link the phenomenon under the other conversion disorders, as dissociative in nature.

Lynn, R. B. and Friedman, L. S. (1995), "Irritable bowel syndrome: Managing the patient with abdominal pain and altered bowel habits", *Medical Clinics of North America*, Vol. 79 (2), pp. 373–90.

Nijenhuis, E. (1999), *Somatoform Dissociation* (Assen, Netherlands: van Gorcum and Co.).

Nijenhuis and his colleagues gave rationale behind the observation that a substantial number of dissociative patients express their dissociativity through somatic, rather than emotional/psychological, symptoms. His somatoform-dissociation questionnaires can be found in the back of his book, or also would be available through the International Society for the Study of Dissociation (ISSD).

Salmon, P., Al-Marzooqi, S. M., Baker, G. and Reilly, J. (2003), "Childhood family dysfunction and associated abuse in patients with nonepileptic seizures: Towards a causal model", *Psychosomatic Medicine*, Vol. 65, pp. 695–700.

The authors tested the hypothesis that a history of sexual abuse is more prevalent in patients with nonepileptic seizures than in controls with epilepsy, that such abuse is a marker of family dysfunction and that the cycle is completed when family dysfunction and abuse are linked to somatization and thus to nonepileptic seizures in some patients.

Talley, N. J. (2002), "Irritable bowel syndrome: A little understood organic bowel disease?", *Lancet*, Vol. 360 (9332), pp. 555–65.

The author, who has written several articles about irritable bowel syndrome over the years, remarks that the disease clusters in families, which he describes as possibly due to intrafamiliar learning and a genetic predisposition. He comments that visceral hypersensitivity is a key feature in most patients, and says that the results of imaging studies of regional cerebral blood flow during rectal distention suggest underlying disturbances of central processing—something that is also seen in other chronic pain syndromes. He comments that treatment "hinges" on an excellent doctor-patient relationship.

Talley, N. J., Boyce, P., and Owen, B. K. (1995), "Psychological distress and seasonal symptom changes in irritable bowel syndrome", *American Journal of Gastroenterology*, Vol. 90 (12), pp. 2115–19.

Thomson, W. G. (1994), "Irritable bowel syndrome: Strategy for the family physician", *Canadian Family Physician*, Vol. 40, pp. 307–16.

Van Dulmen, A. M., Fennis, J. F. M., Mokkink, H. G. A., van der Velden, H. G. M. and Bleijenberg, G. (1994), "Doctors' perception of patients' cognitions and complaints in irritable bowel syndrome at an out-patient clinic", *Journal of Psychosomatic Research*, Vol. 18 (6), pp. 581–90.

One hundred and twenty patients attending an outpatient clinic for functional bowel complaints completed a questionnaire about cognitions regarding their complaints, behavior, and anxiety. Subsequently, doctors completed a similar questionnaire indicating their perceptions of the patients' cognitions, behaviors, and anxiety. Doctors were found to underestimate the patients' expectations and secondary complaints and overestimated the patients' pain-related complaints, catastrophizing, and self-efficacy cognitions. The questionnaire is included in the article.

The final conclusion is that doctors must pay more attention to, and develop the skills for attending to, the patients' complaint-related cognitions and behaviors if therapeutic interventions are to be successful.

Chapter Eight

Diagnostic and Statistical Manual IV (DSM-IV) (1994).

Published by the American Psychiatric Association, this manual gives all the diagnostic criteria for psychiatric and psychological disorders. There has been a revised version since the 1994 edition, and DSM-V is expected to be out in 2005, with a different format, i.e. grouping the "trauma-spectrum" disorders under one heading rather than all over the book.

Van der Kolk, Bessel (1994), "The body keeps the score: Memory and the evolving psychobiology of post-traumatic stress", *Harvard Medical School Psychiatric Review*, pp. 253–65.

Van der Kolk was one of the first, if not the first, to clearly identify that trauma is stored in somatic memory—what was referred to, and dismissed, frequently in the years preceding this excellent article. As always, his reference material is extensive. See also the reference in Chapter Fourteen.

I strongly recommend that every physician read this review. It is easy to find on the Internet, under his name (http://www.trauma-pages.com/vanderk4.htm). Download it and put it in your files. Some articles are never outdated.

Chapter Nine

Felitti, V., Anda R., Nordenberg, D., Williamson, D., Spitz, A., Edwards, V., et al. (1998), "Relationship of childhood abuse and household dysfunction to many of the leading causes of death in adults". *American Journal of Preventive Medicine*, Vol. 14 (4), pp. 245–58.

McFarlane, A. C. (2001), "An overview: Comorbid alcohol abuse or dependence and post-traumatic stress disorder", *American Journal of Psychiatry*, Vol. 158, pp. 1184–90.

Strong, M. (1998), *A Bright Red Scream: Self-Mutilation and the Language of Pain* (Viking Press/Allen Lane).

Van der Kolk, B. A. (2003), "The psychobiology of post-traumatic stress disorder", in Jaak Panksepp (ed.), *Textbook of Biological Psychiatry* (New York, NY: John Wiley & Sons).

Van der Kolk points out that traumatic memories persist mainly in the implicit memory system, often expressed in somatic or behavioral ways, and secondarily as vague, incomplete, and disorganized narratives when put into words. He asks the question, "What keeps the [person] from maintaining [his or her] homeostasis and thus returning to a non-traumatic state?", and goes on to describe the fundamental problem in PTSD as a "fixation on the trauma".

He goes on to describe the psychophysiological effects of trauma, e.g. the heightened arousal syndrome, flashbacks, a failure of the CNS to synthesize the sensations related to the event into a semantic narrative.

Neuroimaging of PTSD patients frequently displays increased amygdala activation in response to traumatic reminders, and the sequelae of this are discussed at length.

Chapter Ten

Van der Kolk, B. A., Pelkovitz, D., Roth, S., Mandel, F. S., McFarlane, M. D. and Herman, J. L. (1996), "Dissociation, affect dysregulation and somatization: The complex nature of adaptation to trauma", invited paper in honor of John Nemiah, *American Journal of Psychiatry*, Vol. 153 (7), Festschrift Supplement, pp. 83–93.

In this lengthy and rich paper, the authors discuss various ways in which individuals adapt to trauma—through PTSD symptomatology, dissociation, somatization and/or affect dysregulation. They feel that these responses must be considered even when the memories of the trauma no longer appear to be intrusive.

Physical problems for which "no cause" can be determined are reflected by a severely disturbed sense of self in several dimensions, such as in being helpless, in being in effective, in being damaged, or in body image.

Further, those who have suffered significant abuse before the age of fourteen years often develop more dissociative problems, anger-management difficulty, self-destructive tendency, and suicidal behaviors than those who were victims at an older age.

The authors also discuss the neurophysiology of trauma with examples of research tools such as positron-emission tomography (PET).

Chapter Eleven

Claude-Pierre, P. (1997), *The Secret Language of Eating Disorders* (Vancouver, B. C.: Random House of Canada).

Peggy Claude-Pierre is the woman who established an internationally known center for the treatment of anorexia, which was eventually closed down because of her intransigence to follow the demands of the Ministry of Children and Families and the Ministry of Health in the province of British Columbia.

This book describes her reasons for setting up the Montreux Clinic—basically, because both her daughters had suffered from anorexia and she, with her dogged persistence, finally got them through it. She has an excellent understanding of the dissociative nature of anorexia (the "secret language") that I believe contributed to her success. However, I take issue with her program of 24-hour watch-dogging, which I think entrenches dependency rather than supporting self-reliance and personal responsibility. There is, however, no question about her dedication to the cause.

Kaplan A. S. and Garfinkle, P. E. (1999), "Difficulties in treating patients with eating disorders: A review of patient and clinician variables", *Canadian Journal of Psychiatry*, Vol. 44 (7), pp. 665–70.

This article recognizes the difficulties associated with treating patients who have eating disorders and points out that the variables include both physician and patient. In the former group are lack of understanding of the biopsychosocial pathophysiology, lack of experience, and countertransference issues. In the second group of variables are the nature of the patients' symptoms, trust issues, and comorbidity.

Kaye, W., et al. (1999), "New directions in treatment research of anorexia and bulimia nervosa", *Biological Psychiatry*, Vol. 45 (10), pp. 1285–92.

The authors point out that response to treatment in these disorders is often poor, and they wonder whether this might be attributed to the fact that, generally, the therapies used have been adopted from those used to treat other psychiatric illnesses. They state, "… eating disorders are independently transmitted familial liabilities with a unique patho-physiology." Obviously, the suggestion is that more understanding of the pathogenesis will bring about improved techniques.

Stoving, R. K., et al. (1999), "A review of endocrine changes in anorexia nervosa", *Journal of Psychiatric Research*, Vol. 33 (2), pp. 139–52.

This review article, done by researchers in Denmark, recognizes that anorexia nervosa is associated with numerous endocrine abnormalities. The syndrome changes hypothalamic monoamines (especially serotonin), neuropeptides (especially neuropeptide Y and cholecystokinin) and leptin, which are all involved in the regulation of human appetite. One of the questions presented is whether the changes in endocrine function are secondary to the eating disorder, or etiologic. The preliminary conclusion was that, at present, none of the abnormalities appear to be primary, but that the probability of a vicious cycle is certainly present.

Watson, T .L., Bowers, W. A. and Andersen, A. E. (2000), "Involuntary treatment of eating disorders", *American Journal of Psychiatry*, Vol. 157 (11), pp. 1806–10.

This article compares the results with patients who were committed (i.e. hospitalized involuntarily) and those who went into the hospital program on a voluntary basis. The conclusion was that the treatment outcomes were the same. (I might say that many of my colleagues would dispute this—the patients are "good little girls" while in hospital but revert immediately to their former eating habits as soon as they are out of the hospital.)

Chapter Twelve

DSM-IV (1994): See Chapter Eight.

Chapter Thirteen

Hunter, M. E. (1995), "Considerations in the treatment of sexual dysfunction in abuse survivors", *Hypnos*, Vol. XXII (2).

This article followed a paper given at the American Society of Clincal Hypnosis Annual Meeting in San Diego. It specifically addresses many of the special needs abuse survivors have, regarding sexual function. Both male and female dysfunction are described, as well as the various somatic symptoms that are most common. Shame and blame are also addressed.

Chapter Fourteen

I have already referred to Daniel Siegel's superb book (see Introduction); in it you will find an excellent description of attachment theory.

Chapter Sixteen

Ainsworth, M. D. S., Blehar, M. C., Waters, E. and Wall, S. (1978), *Patterns of Attachment: A psychological study of the Strange Situation*, (Hillsdale, NJ; Erlbaum).

This is the landmark study which launched a whole new understanding of how early interaction between very small children and their primary caregivers sets the scene for so much future behavior and response. It attends to the importance of what the caregiver experienced when he or she was young, and how that impacted on the ability to connect, emotionally, with that infant and reflect the responses; this in turn, sets the scene for the child developing a sense of trust and security, or lack of it.

Bowlby, J. (1969), *Attachment and Loss*, Vol. I, *Attachment* (New York, NY: Basic Books).

Main, M. and Solomon, J. (1986), "Discovery of an insecure-disor-ganized/disoriented attachment pattern", in T. B. Brazelton and M. Yogman (eds), *Affective Development in Infancy*, (Norwood, NJ; Ablex), pp. 95–124.

The recognition of a fourth (Type D) response in the Strange Situation helps us to understand how early trauma—whatever that type of trauma may be, including emotional—sets the scene for various personality disorders later in life, and opened the way to an understanding of dissociativity.

Main, M. and Morgan, H. (1996), "Disorganization and Dis-orientation in infant Strange Situation behavior: Phenotype resemblance to dissociative states", in L. K. Michelson and W. J. Ray (eds), *Handbook of Dissociation: Theoretical, empirical and clinical perspectives*, (New York, NY: Plenum Press), pp. 107–38.

The "simultaneous contradictory internal working models of Type D attachment" which these authors explore gives us insight into the at times aggravating and bizarre behavior patterns which we see in many of the personality disorders, including borderline personality disorder and the various dissociative disorders. It also paves the way, therefore, to a little more leniency in our response to these patterns, as they confront us in the office, the emergency room or the demands for "unwarranted" time and attention.

Rossi, Ernest (1986), *The Psychobiology of Mind–Body Healing* (New York, NY: W. W. Norton).

Rossi was also a pioneer in linking physiology with somatosen-sory experience and function. This book is particularly focused on hypnotic approaches to healing, but the basic premise is summed up in the final chapter of the book:

> Traditional *psychosomatic symptoms* and, perhaps, most mind-body problems are acquired by a process of experiential learning—specifically, the state-dependent learning of response patterns of Selye's General Adaptation Syndrome. Enduring mind-body problems are manifestations of these state-bound patterns of learning that are encoded within a limbic-hypothalamic system "filter" which modulates mind–body communication.

A new edition of the book came out in 2002. This is another "must" for your bookshelf.

Rossi, Ernest (2002), *The Psychobiology of Gene Expression: Neuroscience and Neurogenesis in Hypnosis and the Healing Arts* (New York, NY: W. W. Norton).

Neurogenesis is Rossi's newest interest. In a lecture given at the European Congress of Hypnosis and Hypnotherapy in Psychosomatic Medicine and Hypnotherapy in Rome in 2002, which I attended, he described the latest theories that nerve and brain cells can, indeed, regenerate. Some of the data included the apparent increase in the volume of the hippocampi of Vietnam veterans, where these structures had shrunk in size due to the severe PTSD and inability to process the experiences from right to left brain. These research studies have been done many decades since the Vietnam war, and until recently the shrunken size had been constant, so regeneration (assuming that this is indeed what happens) obviously took a very long time. The concept of nerve-cell regeneration is very intriguing and opens up many opportunities for exploration and new treatment attitudes and aspects.

Scaer, R. C. (2001), "The neurophysiology of dissociation and chronic disease", *Applied Psychophysiology and Biofeedback*, Vol. 26 (1), pp. 73–94.

In this splendid and extensive article, Scaer describes this work as "… a model of PTSD linked to cyclical autonomic dysfunction, triggered and maintained by the laboratory method of kindling, and perpetuated by increasingly profound dorsal vagal tone and endorphinergic reward systems".

It is a long article but well worth the time and effort to read and to absorb Scaer's message and considerations. It also confirms the hypothesis, presented in this book, that chronic disorders are essentially dissociative in nature. He uses the model of whiplash to validate and exemplify his hypothesis. Painstaking neurophysiological research, explained in detail, confirms his conclusions.

Van der Kolk, B., and van der Hart, Onno (1991), "The intrusive past: The flexibility of memory and the engraving of trauma", *American Imago*, Vol. 48 (4), p. 425.

The authors discuss the importance of a unified memory of experience, and how dismembered fragments of such experience can become fixed ideas and expressions. They describe the role of myelinization in this process, and the state-dependent nature of memory for traumatic events.

Chapter Eighteen

International Society for the Study of Dissociation
60 Revere Dr., Suite 500
Northbrook, IL 60062
Telephone: 847/480-0899 Fax: 847/480-9282
E-mail: issd@issd.org
Website: http://www.issd.org/

Canadian Society for Studies in Trauma and Dissociation
c/o Anne Dietrich
E-mail: amdma@telus.net

U.K. branch of the ISSD:
International Membership Task Force (IMTF)
Rémy Aquarone, Chairman Subcommittee
Pottergate Centre for Dissociation,
26 Princess Street,
Norwich NR3 1AE.
United Kingdom
E-mail: remyaquarone@btconnect.com
Website: http://www.dissociation.co.uk/

Australia:
c/o Dr. Warwick Middleton, Belmont Hospital, Brisbane

Chapter Nineteen

False Memory Syndrome Foundation—information available on the Internet (http://www.fmsfonline.org/).

Herman, J. L. (1992), *Trauma and Recovery* (New York, NY: Basic Books).

Loftus, Elizabeth: Loftus is known for her research in memory and is a spokesperson for the False Memory Syndrome Foundation. Her work is controversial for those who work in the field of trauma and dissociation. She lives in Oregon.

Scheflin, Alan: Scheflin is well known for his clear-sighted presentations of the legal intricacies that accompany work in the dissociative field, as well as the field of clinical hypnosis. His 1989 book *Trance on Trial* (New York, NY: Guildford Press), written with Jerrold Lee Shapiro, is a classic.

Chapter Eighteen
How and When to Refer

As always, we refer a patient when we feel that our understanding of the situation is not sufficient to give the patient the best possible care. However, we also need to be cognizant of what our understanding of any patient's particular situation needs to be.

Seldom is it our job to be the therapist (present writer excepted!). Our job is to keep the patient well, especially physically well, but always aware of the mind–body connection and that what goes on in the one is reflected in the other. In order to so this, we need to understand about dissociative disorders and how they are manifested in any particular patient.

In that role, we care for all aspects of health from birth to death, including assessing the need for surgical intervention, for obstetrical care that is more complex than we feel we can give, for anxieties and depressions, and all the other woes that may afflict the human condition. In other words, for the majority of situations, referral is based on the same criteria as it is with any patient.

However, there are times when we are aware that the patient is dissociative in some degree, that referral needs to be accompanied by rather more explanation than usual, so that the consultant is apprised of the situation and won't be caught off guard.

In my opinion, it is absolutely crucial that these factors be discussed thoroughly with the patient and that we be sensitive to the patient's need, for example, of a woman consultant rather than a man (or vice versa). It may be that you feel your consultant of choice is far and away the best person in the field, and that opinion, and the reasons for it, must be offered to the patient, but the choice is still the prerogative of the patient.

When it comes to psychological or psychiatric referral, the problem is a little more dicey. At the top of the priority scale is the consultant's experience with, and comfort level in, treating dissociative disorders. Assessment is often the first need, so that everybody, patient included, can know where they stand. There are sometimes experts in the field whose main role is to provide such assessments, but who may not wish to undertake the role of psychotherapist. That should be made clear to the patient at the outset, so that he understands that this particular consultant may not end up being the therapist. Or the patient may be interested in the assessment, but not be ready to enter into therapy at that time.

How to find the right consultant

Contact your local branch of the International Society for the Study of Dissociation (ISSD), or any of its component societies in other countries. If there is no such resource available, often the Section of Psychiatry of the Medical Association in your state, province or district may be able to give you the names of two or three psychiatrists who are knowledgeable. The same goes for psychologists or registered clinical counselors: consult with the College of Psychologists or its equivalent where you live. They are almost always aware of the subspecialties of their members.

We all need the help of specialists when we find ourselves out of our depth. That's what the specialists are for, after all. Usually, after the presenting situation is diagnosed and advice given, we then undertake the continuing care of the patient. That is not usually the case with these disorders (nor would we want it to be). But it *is* very important to keep an ongoing connection between physician and psychotherapist, with the patient's full consent. Otherwise, important details that are crucial to the overall health of the patient may slip through the cracks.

One more thing: our staff also need to understand what is going on. All too often, when the patient calls while in an angry or depressed or demanding mood, the staff tend to find it difficult to maintain a smile in their voices. It's understandable. They are the ones who have to cope with the demands, after all, and somehow placate the patient until the doctor can take over. Just a better awareness of what dissociation-DID, DDNOS, or PTSD—is all about will often solve the matter.

I trust you will find, as I have, that seldom do we meet patients who are more needy, demanding, hard working, exasperating, determined to get well, difficult to get along with, or creative than those who are dissociative. I have learned far more about the art, not just the science, of medicine from those struggling, often suffering, and courageous people, than from any other group of patients in all the years of my practice of medicine. I honor them, and thank them for teaching me so much about what otherwise I never would have known.

Chapter Nineteen
Changes in the Field

It has been more than a quarter of a century since that bewildering year when I first found myself flummoxed, looking for ways to figure out this really pleasant and interesting—and frustrating— new patient whom I had acquired from the colleague who was moving to another city. Looking back, I realize I made so many mistakes that I marvel how my patients, in those early days, were so patient with me! Until the advent of the First International Conference on Multiple Personality and Dissociation in 1983, there was so little help to be had and we were all struggling along independently, hoping that we were doing the right things. I've written about the overwhelming joy when we found all those other therapists who had been struggling too! We gritted our teeth and plunged on, still hoping that we were doing the best for our patients; the wonderful part was that our patients knew this, and so were more than willing to teach us as we journeyed together across a very unfamiliar and rocky emotional and psychological moonscape.

After a few years, we thought that we really understood. We knew some of the approaches that were absolutely essential to good therapy, and learned how to use them. Little did we know how the field would change in the next two decades, thanks to that sophisticated and elegant research to which I have previously referred.

This final chapter in the book is simply to point out a few of the changes in the field, in areas where we pretty well thought we had it made.

Use of hypnosis

As I remember it, almost all of us felt that the use of hypnosis was mandatory if we were to help the patient break through amnesic barriers and retrieve their memories of abuse—a process that we also felt was mandatory.

It took me some time to realize that, although virtually all dissociative patients were hypnotic virtuosos (to quote a friend of mine), some of them were not happy about deliberately using it in therapy. In time I realized that it was just too reminiscent of what they did to distance themselves from the abuse while it was happening.

Nevertheless, I worked diligently to persuade them that it would be for the best—at least I did that until I had coped with one abreaction too many in the office and realized that, while hypnosis was a great tool for many people, including many dissociative patients, it wasn't the tool of choice for some. I found that other therapists were having some of the same experiences and making the same changes in their techniques.

So I began to be much more judicious in my use of hypnosis with dissociative patients. I found it was great for teaching ego-strengthening techniques, problem-solving gimmicks, self-hypnosis and relaxation, ways to improve sleep patterns and to rehearse difficult situations such as applying for a job or going to the dentist, but I stopped "trying" to help the patient "get the memories back".

Does it sometimes facilitate the process of sorting out memories? Yes, of course, sometimes it can and does. But, as I will describe in the next section, there are ways to organize that in order to make it even more useful.

Understanding memory

Ah, if we only had that little video camera that we used to believe was tucked securely away somewhere in the subconscious depths of our brains! Instead, we now have to accept the fact that memory is infinitely malleable; that what happens to us one day is never remembered exactly the way it really happened, even a day or so later, and certainly not years later. It's as if we were a micro-example of the very true adage that two people, watching the same scene, will invariably describe it somewhat differently. Siblings have been known to argue hotly about what one remembers happened one way, and the other remembers it as if it happened on Mars. In dissociative disorders, however, it is two or more parts of the self who remember it in those various ways. And it is also true that, although explicit memory is often very inaccurate and subject to what some theorists call "decay", implicit memory is thought by those same theorists to be extremely resistant to decay, especially when it involved highly emotional responses.

The terms "implicit memory" and "explicit memory" were unknown in those early years. We did understand that traumatic memories were processed differently than other memories, and we conjectured that that was because of the hormonal flooding that occurred with trauma, which is true. But "implicit" and "explicit" were not in the usual memory vocabulary for most of us.

Once we learned about it, however, the difference began to make such sense. Paying attention with the cognitive brain during traumatic situations, or when we were younger than two years of age, or somehow deliberately transmogrifying those situations from cognition into body memories? Nonsense.

However, realizing the difference between narrative, logical memory where we pay attention and talk about it, and experiential memory, to which we seldom pay the same sort of attention and do not talk about it in the same way, and recognizing that these two different kinds of memory are even stored in different parts of the brain, depending on hippocampal processing—now *that* makes sense.

Through the years it became very clear to me that there is no need to go digging for memories. They will come when it is time, when the person is ready, at a deep level, to start remembering. In fact, when it is time, you can't really stop them.

We also began to realize how useful it could be to fractionate the remembering process—as was elegantly described by Dr.

181

Catherine Fine. One doesn't have to be submerged by the flood of memory: we can "push the pause button" (my way of describing it) and release it again when we are ready to continue. That could be in a few minutes, or after a few weeks.

I found that my patients were able to tell me, and felt good about telling me, that "something's brewing and it's just about ready to come out". So we would set up the appointment, as I have said before, at the end of the office day when the waiting room is cleared. A lot of work was accomplished that way. It also may be useful to video the remembering process, or "abreaction", and use it to debrief later.

This is probably not the sort of work that you are going to be doing, but it's interesting to know about, I think. It is also entirely possible to establish the length of time set aside for sessions, including memory-retrieval sessions. You may want to remember this when you are establishing boundaries and limits for patient visits to your office.

Never "lead the witness"

This also has to do with the retrieval of memories, and with the whole "false-memory syndrome" that sprang up in the early 1990s.

I am not a supporter of the False Memory Syndrome Foundation, which I believe has brought infinitely more pain to those who were already suffering dreadfully. But I do understand the anguish of parents who believed themselves to be falsely accused. Unfortunately, many well-meaning therapists *did* help their patients to go digging for the memories, and also "led the witness" as those experiential excavations continued. "Who else is there?" implies that there is someone else there. "What does he look like?" implies that there is a person and it is a male. It's not hard to understand the evolution of hundreds of court cases. Unfortunately, it also caused many excellent therapists, diligent and honest in their work, to break under the undeserved load of lawsuits on their backs.

We know better now, understanding that our role is to bear witness, as Judith Herman says in her wonderful book, *Trauma and Recovery*, and to "be there" for our patients as they struggle on. And so I put into practice the wise words of my colleague Dr. Claire Frederick, and offer "helpful noises": "Mmmm"; "Ah"; "Yes, I'm here"; "Umhumm"; and so on. My patients know that I have not deserted and will not desert them, but they also understand that it is *their* journey, and not mine, and it is my job to help them find *their* truth, and not mine.

FMS also did one wonderful thing for the field of dissociation: it forced us to do the research, to gather the psychoneurological data to support, clarify, amend, or discard our old theories. We should be grateful.

Emphasis on professional training

It seems supremely ironic that I, a family physician who learned about the treatment of dissociative disorders by the seat of my pants, so to speak, should be such a strong advocate for professional training for therapists in the field. In my own defense, however, I did go to all the courses I could find (not many, in those early years, and almost all at clinical hypnosis meetings), conferred and still confer with dozens of professional colleagues, and read, read, read whenever any new book or paper or journal came out. And I, who detested neurophysiology in medical school, now find it absolutely fascinating. One never knows how or when life is going to throw an unexpected curve—even a helpful one.

We need training if we are to be useful and not harmful for our patients. That is why I wrote this book. Certainly, I was never taught about dissociative disorders in medical school, and I doubt that there are many medical schools where it is taught, even now—certainly not in family medicine. And yet, and yet—we really are the sentinels, and we must learn how to carry out that obligation in the very best way we can.

Index